MEDICATION DETOX

MEDICATION
DETOX

HOW TO LIVE
YOUR BEST HEALTH

RACHEL REINHART
TAYLOR, MD

NEW YORK

LONDON • NASHVILLE • MELBOURNE • VANCOUVER

MEDICATION DETOX
HOW TO LIVE YOUR BEST HEALTH

© 2021 RACHEL REINHART TAYLOR, MD

Published in New York, New York, by Morgan James Publishing in partnership with Difference Press. Morgan James is a trademark of Morgan James, LLC. www.MorganJamesPublishing.com

ISBN 978-1-64279-941-5 paperback
ISBN 978-1-64279-942-2 eBook
ISBN 978-1-64279-943-9 Audio
Library of Congress Control Number: 2019919328

Cover Design Concept:
Nakita Duncan

Cover Design:
Rachel Lopez
www.r2cdesign.com

Editor:
Bethany Davis

Book Coaching:
The Author Incubator

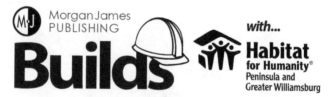

Morgan James is a proud partner of Habitat for Humanity Peninsula and Greater Williamsburg. Partners in building since 2006.

Get involved today! Visit
www.MorganJamesBuilds.com

For my daughter Delilah,
who believed in me even when I didn't.

TABLE OF CONTENTS

FOREWORD

As a long-time certified Transformational Meditation facilitator and life-coach I'm honored to offer some insight as to why this book is both life-changing and saving.

Medication Detox by Dr. Taylor is a ray of sunshine in a dark place. So many want to believe that their physical issues are only treatable by medication because taking some personal responsibility for becoming well again is too difficult. Dr. Taylor does an amazing job of breaking down what *responsibility* looks like in action. And, when you read about how she has overcome her own "illnesses" through first, just self-awareness and reflection, you will understand how it is possible for you to get off the meds and feel happy, healthy, and whole again.

This book is like having a generational family doctor who knows your mental, physical, and emotional states well enough to suggest a plan for your success based on the healthiest outcome possible. Wisely, Dr. Taylor never suggests that western medicine practices are bad or not good for you. Instead, she blends her extensive western training with proven non-traditional techniques learned through self- discovery and years spent in the Native American communities that achieve lasting success. She is to medicine, what fabled Robin Hood was to money. I'd call her a modern-day Rachel Hood, a person committed to making sure everyone can afford to walk their unique path to healthy living.

If you're actually ready to put blame aside and begin taking just a few of the ever so many steps she offers for healing in this book, you can be successful in your desires for happy and healthy again—without negative side effects.

I believe the best part of "Medication Detox" is that she has so much empathy and passion for helping you. You can literally hear it in every chapter. And, every chapter offers another approach and steps to wellness that you may have *known* but never really thought possible for you. These approaches are not a fix but as the title says, an effective and lasting detox that can be as aggressive or gradual as you like. She speaks to the parts of you that are ready to be healed and shows the way. Your best health is a simple plan of action, created by you, with her direction.

I have been blessed to spend time with Dr. Rachel Reinhart Taylor and can speak with confidence in telling you she is the real deal, a person with a big heart, and even bigger knowledge of how to get you healthy again so you can enjoy life. Allow her desire to be your desire, and watch the miracles unfold.

I wish you well in this wonderful adventure.

—**Ell Graniel**, Best Selling Author of *Get Happier, Fitter, & Off the Meds Now: 7 Steps to Improved Health and a Body You Love* and, *Chocolate Cake for the Thighs: The Anti Diet Book for Women*

CHAPTER 1

WHAT IS YOUR CHRONIC DISEASE COSTING YOU?

"Insanity is doing the same thing over and over and expecting different results."
—Albert Einstein

I remember sitting in my primary care doctor's office and hearing yet another new diagnosis. Another thing I believed I was going to deal with for the rest of my life. My heart sank; how was I going to manage paying for everything that came with it? The cost of the medications, the new specialist I would have to go see, the imaging studies, the treatment. Now I had another thing that was going to keep me from enjoying time with my family and friends, another thing that made me different, another problem. And how was I going to schedule my work to go to these appointments? I wasn't really allowed to take time off during the day as they could need me any time, and if I was gone an actual life could be in danger. There was nobody to cover for me, as we were short-staffed as it was. The worries built up quickly and caused almost constant stress and an overwhelmed feeling at the inability to fit everything into my life. As a physician myself, I knew that I was becoming a "complicated patient" and wondered how it came to this.

You too might know this feeling, or something similar, when diagnosed with any sort of disease, even if you feel it is inevitable. Being healthy becomes a full-time job. You may suffer through severe side effects (such as diarrhea, headache, exhaustion, weight gain, nutritional deficiencies causing numbness in legs and feet, dehydration, and pain) just to be able to control the advance of the disease, just as I did, because you do not know you have another option. Or perhaps because the other options seem insurmountable and you don't believe that you can, in fact, make the changes in lifestyle necessary to reverse your disease.

You may believe, as I did, that your disease is not reversible. That you now have something that will never go away and will continue to get worse regardless of what you do. I will tell you a secret: diseases pretty much all are reversible if you give your body a chance. Sometimes the medications we take cause us to need more medications and have even more "diseases" when really what we're experiencing are actually just medication side effects!

So how do I know? As a doctor I used to believe that a lot of chronic illnesses are permanent, like most of my colleagues do, but research is increasingly pointing at lifestyle being the root cause of disease, and medication side effects being another component— even when you think you're experiencing a new disease!

How did I reverse my own and my patients' chronic diseases? It wasn't how I thought I was going to do it, but it started with changing inside. It may sound very cliché, but the secret to how I started reversing disease and coming off the medications is in the following pages. Even in the cases of diseases I didn't *think* were reversible, I have been pleasantly surprised at my improvement since applying these new habits

We may not even know that the lifestyle choices we are making are causing a disease. We might even think we are doing something "good" for our bodies. At some point everybody has believed they were doing something great that science has later found was not at all good for you. More often than not it involves buying something to put on/in your body. If I could have titled this book in fancy medical terms, it would be called *Exogenous Substance Detox*, meaning detoxing from *anything* not originating inside your body. That includes medications, supplements, juices, "cleanses," herbal products, spices, drugs and alcohol, excessive exercise, and—I like to add—"other people's advice." There are a few caveats to that obviously: we need food and water to live (we will get into that later).

If you don't think all this is a big deal and you don't want to improve, that's up to you. If you don't think it's costing you much, here are some fancy studies. The cost of almost every chronic disease is astronomical. According to the National Association of Chronic Disease Directors, "Health care costs for people with a chronic condition average $6,032 annually—five times higher than for those without such a condition."[1] These are all reversible. Although this can be said about almost any chronic disease, I will give as an example:3` the cost of one of the most common reversible diseases—type 2 diabetes (adult diabetes). On the American Diabetes Association website, the statistic for the cost of having type 2 diabetes is staggering, about $9,601 per year. This a reversible and completely avoidable disease that can wreak havoc on a person's life.[2]

You may end up not only feeling like your health is out of your control, but also having severe psychological consequences due to things like the stress and worry created from having to manage your disease—keeping track of things like taking medications, hospitalizations, doctor visits, lab tests, and feeling that it getting worse is "inevitable." Then what can sometimes feel even worse is the social stigma. Your self-worth deteriorates, and you can be left with feelings of worthlessness and even sometimes severe depression. You might even blame yourself for your disease, causing a destructive cycle of self-deprecation. How do I know this? Not only because I have been the primary care doctor for some of these good people who beat themselves up despite doing their best, but because I was that patient, too. Even as a physician I believed I was severely flawed because of my own physical and mental health, and it took close to a miracle to realize I had fallen down the rabbit hole that I had helped so many patients climb back out of.

What causes this spiraling into such self-doubt and insecurity because of chronic illness? I believe that the majority of it comes from our environment. Not just our family or our own unique situations, but I believe there is a bigger, more pervasive problem that reaches all homes, regardless of money or status. When remedied it creates a whole person who is able to make their own decisions and take back their health. In my own personal experience, when I started fixing this everything else, including clarity about how to treat and reverse my own chronic physical and mental illness, improved.

What is this problem that, if resolved, can create an overall improved life and health? It is this: insecurity. I know, you don't think you're insecure, because you're taught it's not *okay* to be insecure. Your insecurity is not your fault, though. Here's why.

Insecurity is an almost global phenomenon and is not just due to our own weakness. As a matter of fact, I think that individual people are almost never to blame. Let me explain with an example. I was at a car dealership having the taillight on my car fixed. As I was waiting there, I walked around a bit looking at the posters on the wall. On one of the posters there was a very handsome man standing next to a fancy car in the snow. In big red letters there were the words: CHOOSE CONFIDENCE THIS WINTER, GET A WINTER PACKAGE. I almost burst out laughing as I thought to myself, *Wow, they are really digging at all of our insecurity,* but then I started to think about how many people have probably decided they should get the winter package from this poster. Not because they needed it, but because buying it would improve their confidence (or so they thought). Though I'm sure few would like to admit it, surely this advertisement has been successful because of the general population's insecurity.

For a long time I was, and still am sometimes, insecure and unsure of myself, which I think is quite normal for our environment. What do I mean by this? I mean, think about how most people make their money: by selling something. This can range from a product to entertainment to medications to appointments…anything you can charge money for, I'm sure somebody has sold (or will sell). Selling things is almost always based on convincing somebody that they are not whole without it. Let me say that again: *Selling things is almost always based on convincing somebody that they are not whole without it.* Of course we walk around being inundated with ads that our conscious and subconscious pick up and absorb. These ads tell us we aren't good enough, without us even agreeing to watch the ad or knowing we did it. They are all over the internet, TV, and social media, whether we know they are there or not. While I don't think anything is wrong with getting paid for your work, the marketing is getting out of control. This is something I thought I knew that was driven home when I learned about the "Pink Tax."

The Pink Tax is basically an upcharge for products for women that are almost the same as a man's product but somehow cost more. For example, disposable razors. The cute, pink girl version of a disposable razor will cost about 20% more than a razor made for a man by the same company with almost the same exact features. A common marketing scheme is "shrink it and pink it," meaning appeal to women by making something cuter and then charge them more.

I have to admit that this has worked on me many, many times. When I started seeing more clearly all the things I had bought into, I beat *myself* up because I thought about how dumb I must have been to buy into them. In reality, advertisers know exactly what they're doing and keep doing it! Then they get the general population to feel like somehow they are the ones who are wrong if they don't agree with them.

Our whole society is being told all the time in subtle ways that we are wrong and incomplete. Our subconscious mind walks around absorbing images and advertisements that play in the background while we aren't even paying attention. These advertisements love to tell us how in some way we are not a whole person and if we don't buy whatever they are selling, we are going to continue to be unhappy forever. Of course nobody wants to tell us that we are perfect exactly as we are. How would their business be successful if they did? With few exceptions, this has become the norm and is now accepted by most.

Unfortunately, Western medicine, too, has become mostly a business. While, in my experience, most Western medicine doctors want to make a human connection with their patients, get to know them, and encourage them, the pressures of the business of medicine have become overwhelming. Ads on television for medications also lead people to believe that their problems are terrible, and the only way to solve them and be happy is to take drastic measures. Some of the side effects commonly mentioned in ads are not well discussed and can actually end up leading to death.

For example, I see ads for people with skin diseases like psoriasis. I know this can be quite detrimental, create self-consciousness on a patient's part, and lead to other diseases if not controlled. However, the ads show somebody cowering in the corner looking heartbroken and lost, a feeling we may have all experienced before. Then they show the patient after taking the medication: happy, in the sunshine, participating in a sport or having fun with family, etc. They don't detail that there are way less drastic options or that the medication suppresses your immune system. Suppression of your immune system can quickly lead to infections that an otherwise healthy body would fight off, but without the immune system can cause death. But the ad promises happiness, and you want that happiness. We understand that; we all want happiness.

Primary care doctors are in high demand since the "art" of medicine has become a business that drives them out of practice. Primary care doctors are not paid what they bill; as a matter of fact, we will be lucky to see twenty-five percent of that. The cost of keeping a clinic open—paying staff, medications, insurance, licensure—is far more than that of most businesses. Doctors become forced to push patients through quickly to be able to keep their doors open in a way that none of us ever wanted when we started. In addition, for the amount of time we spend with each patient, there will be double that in charting/writing notes/follow-up. So, if on a regular day I'm at the clinic eight hours and see three patients per hour (without any breaks) I will see twenty-four patients. If I spend ten minutes with each patient then I will have twenty more minutes of work per patient, which comes to 480 minutes (eight hours) of work *after* I see a patient. So if I see patients for four hours (ten minutes each) and spend eight more hours that day charting, checking labs results, refilling medications, getting prior authorization etc., that's a twelve-hour day, at least five days a week.

Physicians never go home and forget about work, though; they get contacted all day and night all week, varying based on their practice. This also does not include all the extra requirements placed on physicians that almost no other business calls for. These include extraordinary amounts of time and money paid to keep up with numerous licenses, boards, credentials, and registrations required to practice. I *want* to spend time getting to know, connecting with, and helping every patient, but if I did that (and owned my own clinic) my business would not stay open no matter how much I love my patients. As a patient, I've even been to a primary care doctor so inundated with tasks that he didn't look at me once our entire appointment and forgot to do a physical exam until I reminded him! I was annoyed at first, as any patient would be, but *completely understood* because the business of it is overwhelming, despite most physicians just at heart wanting to help others. Also, it is almost impossible for physicians to take last-minute days off for emergencies, which can compound the stress and distraction throughout each day because we are still human beings as well.

The point I'm making is that we are all human beings doing our best so let's give ourselves a break. When we don't believe in ourselves and know that we are perfect as we are, things become worse. This goes for everything from outer appearance to chronic disease. I had to finally stop and look at what was going on inside of me and work on it. Though I did not expect the result to be overturning diagnoses I'd had for over ten years, that was one of the many pleasant surprises. Once I made these changes for myself, I started realizing that what I had done in the past to help patients get off medications and reverse their diseases wasn't just mindlessly throwing recommendations at them. I had helped them believe in themselves. They started changing how they saw themselves on the inside, creating a cascade of overall life improvement and reversal of disease. They simplified their lives and lived their best health as I had done. In time, this became the catalyst to reverse disease and simplify their lives to better health.

CHAPTER 2

DOCTORS ARE PEOPLE TOO

"The reward for conformity is that everyone likes you except for yourself."
– Rita Mae Brown

octors have the highest suicide rate of any profession. In 2018, studies showed that one doctor commits suicide in the United States every day, or 40 suicides per 100,000 doctors. To put that into perspective, the average suicide rate of the general population is 12.3 suicides per 100,000 people. I could have been a part of that statistic and personally knew two doctors that are.

Let's start at the beginning. Before we do though, I want to make it very clear that this part is not to blame somebody else, as I truly believe that most people are doing their best, including myself. Unfortunately, we all fall victim to the most common chronic disease—being human.

The mind-body connection is being increasingly proven to be the underlying cause for chronic disease. Emotions that put our bodies on "high alert" are especially taxing, but almost any prolonged state of intense emotion can be taxing if not addressed. Here is my story about how my chronic disease began.

My first memory as a child was feeling a need to comfort my crying mother. She was the single mother of four after my parents divorced when I was around two years old. I cannot imagine how difficult that time was for my mother. We created a strong bond and my mother would refer to me as her "little buddy." As I grew, I remember doing everything I could to include everybody. My mother would tell me how my teachers would tell her that I would be sure to include every single child, especially those who were new at school. Per my recollection, this was a relatively happy time where I did a lot of kid stuff in our small northern Utah town.

When I was around eleven, I came home early from visiting my father to find my mother standing in the living room, beaming from ear to ear. She turned to me and said, "I was going to wait for everybody to get home but I can't wait—look!" She held out her left hand and showed me a diamond ring on her ring finger. She had gotten married after three months of online dating and, from what I understood, her first time meeting her new husband. I was so confused! She went on, "He lives in California and we will be moving there in a month."

I was truly excited for my mother because all this time, since my earliest memory, I had believed my job was to make everybody else, including my mother, happy. I wrote a letter to my new stepfather complete with crayon-drawn pictures telling him how excited I was to meet him. I found out that he had three kids, two girls and a boy, and one of the girls was close to my age. So one month later this new man flew out and helped us pack up the house, and off we all went off to California.

This is where things went horribly wrong. At first things were fun. We had a new dog and a pool to play in. But my excitement about moving to California quickly dissipated into sadness and worry. From my viewpoint, I believed that my mother's happiness was dependent on me and I took on the role of her protector. My stepfather would frequently yell at her and I would stand up to him, saying, "Stop yelling at my mother," to which he would reply, "Shut up Rachel, this is none of your business." My mother just sat there quietly, as did my other siblings. I remember crying almost every night of seventh grade. I remember only rarely did anybody come in to comfort me, and I felt misunderstood.

I vividly remember one occasion when my stepfather became so angry that my mother was worried for our safety and took us over to a neighbor's house. I was terrified as we went back to the house after a couple of hours, but everybody acted like nothing happened. Around the same time, I also remember being alone in a room with my stepfather and crying because I missed my friends and family back home. He looked up and screamed profanities at me while he slapped a stapler off the table, narrowly missing me. My mother didn't seem to do anything, at least not in front of me. I felt deep sadness and horribly alone and that's when I learned to be quiet and suppress all my emotions. If I cried, I got teased, now not only by my brothers but my new stepsiblings. I became more terrified without any healthy outlet. I started "learning" that I was the problem, always. My sympathetic nervous system was on overdrive, I was sleeping poorly, and I was so anxious. I felt abandoned by all those I had taken so much care to show love to, a theme that continued throughout my life. Around that time I began having severe spasms on the right side of my back that were unexplained by any scan or test.

As I entered high school, I joined sports and continued to excel academically, but felt scared at home almost all the time. I was on eggshells around my stepfather, sometimes yelling back, sometimes just hiding. I equated success on paper to love, and so I set out to achieve everything I could to feel what I thought was love and support, if only fleetingly. I wanted to get out of there and my father, still living in Utah, had found an option. It was called "early college," where I completed whatever high school classes I had left to finish at the college and retroactively added them to complete my actual high school diploma. My parents agreed to this, so at age sixteen, after my junior year, I moved back to Utah to start college.

I found this new environment to be extremely focused on what we thought of people's outer appearance, possessions, actions, and what they might think of us if they found out we were not perfect. Having emotions was also not allowed here. It didn't matter anyway, because by now my emotions were so deep and suppressed that I didn't even know they were there, causing chronic release of stress hormones.

For the next few years I continued to try to figure out how to be what I thought my family wanted me to be without having emotions. I spent my college years taking large class loads with an emphasis on getting honors, working sometimes *more* than full time, still trying to overachieve. One of my brothers told me, "Slow down, you're making the rest of us look bad," and now overachieving was taken out of the equation for love. I was trying to figure out how to achieve enough for my parents' approval but not so much my siblings disliked me. My sleep started suffering and life was a whirlwind of doing things I thought my family wanted me to do for their approval. I couldn't help but feel like a constant disappointment, despite getting excellent grades, working more than full time, and having many other talents. I was so lucky to have some great friends in college who I was able to still have fun and let go of the stress with.

I had been accepted to medical school and was preparing to start in the fall. I had had a boyfriend at the time for four months and, despite using birth control, became pregnant. I was pregnant and about to start medical school, and my parents were alluding to my being pregnant out of wedlock and how ashamed they were in many, many ways. In one less subtle comment, my father stated, "What will people think of you if you are pregnant and not married in medical school?" Finally, wanting validation and acceptance, I got married. As medical school started, I studied long hours and my husband at the time was unhappy with his life for various reasons. I didn't drink at all during my pregnancy, but my husband's drinking became heavier and arguments ensued. He would get angry if I had any knowledge that he didn't have and would yell at me, saying, "Oh, you think you're *so* smart" when I needed to study for an exam.

The baby came and things continued about as expected for an arguing couple who now had a new stressor. He would drink, scream, throw things, and then "forget." I was, again, in the same kind of relationship as I had been with my stepfather. I became more scared as he became more threatening. I was exhausted and stressed out. I wanted to leave, but didn't want to disappoint my family. I couldn't sleep, I was agitated, I would cry in frustration. I was never asked if I felt safe at home but instead was diagnosed with post-partum depression. Here's where the medications started—I was put on a low dose of anti-depressants, which worked wonderfully at first. However, as things escalated my dose was doubled, ultimately making me *more* anxious and agitated, after which I slept even less. Because the high dose of anti-depressants created more agitation, the obstetrician who was treating me assumed this meant I was bipolar. It didn't seem to cross anybody's mind, including my own, that perhaps my body was exquisitely sensitive to medication and this was a side effect. I was referred to a psychiatrist, who diagnosed me as bipolar, *again*, without asking me what was going on in my life or if I felt safe at home. I would hope he would have changed his mind had he known the truth, but regardless this started me down a path of many, many Western medications. I could not tolerate them at even low doses, and detrimental side effects seemed to be far more prevalent than the beneficial effects. Other medications were added on to counteract the issues from the first, and at one point I was on thirteen medications per day—only three for my emotions and the rest to counterbalance the side effects.

When I was diagnosed, there was no actual test to confirm bipolar disorder. Psychiatrists would try medication after medication trying to balance each of them out to create emotional balance, forgetting that sometimes the problems may be being created by the first medication.

I think there are absolutely times for medications, at least temporarily, while figuring out what's underneath. Even if you're taking a medication for your whole life, nothing is wrong with a medication that helps make life easier if it's well tolerated and you know the side effects and are willing to experience them. I think it is absolutely warranted to give medications if otherwise you are risking your own and/or others' safety. Thank goodness for medications and procedures when lives are at risk! However, I also know now that when we are quick to put on and permanently leave medications, that may be creating more problems. I believe this is due primarily to the human body having so many functions that we don't understand yet that we can't anticipate every unique side effect for every unique person. Several times over the course of ten years, a new psychiatrist would see me and question if I was really bipolar. I was too scared to be taken off the medications during medical school or my residency, because I was afraid of having feelings again.

Feelings, even normal ones, were not encouraged, especially as a doctor. After a patient dies in my care despite my doing everything according to guidelines, I am taught to suppress my feelings because there is still work to be done and people are waiting to be seen. I doubt that any doctor adequately expresses and heals the emotional pain that is part of the job. In hindsight, what I was doing was taking short-acting medications in small doses that would sedate and suppress emotions. When these medications wore off, then all the feelings that had built up that I had refused to feel in the past came back with a force I was so afraid to feel that I took more medicine to push them back down. This happened a couple of times a day.

After the abusive relationship with my now ex-husband, he convinced me that because I was now labeled as "bipolar," I was not a good mother. He reiterated to me on several occasions that I "drove him to drink" and I believed him. I thought I was a terrible mother and that my daughter would be better off with him. My belief was that I was the problem and that if I was removed from the situation he would become a wonderful human being and father. So, I gave him primary custody. I regretted that decision so many times over the years and continued to believe his emotional abuse. About two years later, I was finally diagnosed with hypothyroidism, or low thyroid. This can be caused for several poorly understood reasons after childbirth and could certainly explain my "postpartum depression," but was tossed aside as the possible reason for the misdiagnosis. Also, one of the medications I had been started on for bipolar disorder was known to be "thyrotoxic," meaning it causes hypothyroidism (low thyroid). Who knows which came first, the medication or the thyroid problem. I was medicated and my mood became much better, but it was too late. I was still treated like somehow my mind and body were separate. The low thyroid was not taken into account by my psychiatrists for years.

Eventually, I graduated from medical school and left to start a surgical residency in Baltimore in 2011. With some concoction of medication mix I set out to start, but was not anticipating the months of wait it would take for me to even get an appointment with a new psychiatrist. One of the medications I took as-needed for anxiety is now known to cause "rebound anxiety," or worsened anxiety when it wears off. This caused me to be stuck in a cycle of "needing" a medication that actually created the anxiety to begin with. This was not something I knew at the time.

I was always on extremely low doses of medications that were poorly tolerated or made me so tired that I fell asleep standing up. Instead of just taking me off my medication, doctors would switch it for something else with almost the same result. My misdiagnosed bipolar disorder had never interfered with my ability to care for patients, I was never hospitalized, and I always took my medications as prescribed from the time I was diagnosed (some of the clues over time that were good evidence that I was not, in fact, bipolar). And my unique relationship with my feelings was beneficial during my residency. I loved connecting with people when I had the chance and I took time to listen, discuss, and respect the opinions and feelings of my patients. I was frequently criticized for having feelings by the same doctors who would ask me to smooth things over with patients whose feelings they had hurt. So I continued to push any feelings down that manifested as physical symptoms.

It is now well documented that things like stress and history of trauma can create chronic abdominal pain and associated symptoms, which I began having. I had repeat stomach pain that led to things like severe nausea and constipation without any "real" reason, meaning scans and tests were negative. I started using laxatives and nausea medications, because taking time off in any residency for illness is basically a hilarious joke. The motto is "You're either a patient in the ER dying, or you're working your shift in the hospital." In my surgical rotation in medical school there was something called the "cry chair." This was not in a kind/safe space way. It was in a berating and making fun of feelings way. I was certainly warned against crying anytime and anywhere—anyone who cried would be the butt of a joke that the whole surgery program would know immediately. So now I was having intermittent palpitations, back and neck spasms worsening due to standing long hours and looking down in the operating room, and abdominal pain with nausea and constipation, while taking a surplus of medications designed to make me "not feel" under a misdiagnosis.

I missed my daughter desperately, but when you apply for residency you don't get options for where you go. There's one day when everybody opens their email and it says, "You go here or nowhere." This was the first time I had moved away from my daughter, and I was regularly met with messages about how I "abandoned my child" and what a terrible mother and person I was. I would ask to talk to her whenever I was free and was frequently told it was not a good time. I tried connecting with my family, but was met with, "Are you taking your medications?" and reactions blaming my "bipolar." I always was taking my medications, of course, but my family kept clinging to a false diagnosis so they could be absolved of any fault for my "emotional nature." I kept believing there was something wrong with me, when really it was the lack of emotion from the people I relied on for support that was the problem. I learned later that this had been discovered to be very closely linked to symptoms similar to bipolar disorder. It's called "emotional neglect" and is nothing to scoff at.

I wanted to push down any feelings even more. I should not have been surprised, but eventually my family began talking to me less and less because my struggle was "uncomfortable" for them. My mother intentionally stopped taking my calls or returning them. I didn't find out until about three years later that it was because she "didn't know what to do" so her solution was to ignore me. There are many studies about trauma and emotional support. One study[3] found that those with no support are prone to post-traumatic stress disorder. Those who had good support were less likely to get it and more likely to have hope and resilience. In hindsight I wonder what would have happened had I had felt supported. I do know that when I *have* been supported during other times of trauma, I was much more easily able to push through them.

Ten years later I have found my low thyroid is being reversed just by coming off the medications that contributed to it, in addition to improving my diet and sleep. I decided to take a break and left my residency, as I felt I was on the edge of breakdown and couldn't bear the thought of how I would look to others. I excavated some of the stress and pain of residency in counseling and started feeling much, much better. However, I still believed that I was the problem when it came to my whole family for basically my entire life. I did notice my chronic abdominal pain with nausea was now gone. I was happier and healthier already. I completed another surgery year in another location without problems and actually enjoyed it! However, I decided that to spend more time with my daughter

I would have to change to a specialty with at least a hope of better hours, family medicine.

I created a relationship with a psychiatrist and therapist in Phoenix where I was to undergo my family medicine residency. Both of them questioned my bipolar disorder diagnosis, and actually I was the one who was still so afraid to feel that I insisted it must be accurate. I kept going with the stress of keeping any and all emotions at bay because I believed this was how people were supposed to act. I pushed down feeling after feeling and eventually started having migraines on top of all the previously mentioned issues. These began with part of my vision becoming blurry and then, about twenty minutes later, the severe head pain, sensitivity to lights, and vomiting began. My migraines became more and more frequent, to the point where I was getting Botox injections in the back of my head and neck (not for cosmetic purposes in my face—I wish it was a choice like that) every three months. As soon as the blurred vision would start, I would take several medications in the hopes I could avoid the oncoming migraine and continue with work.

Over time though, my migraines continued to worsen. I graduated from residency and started my job in the emergency rooms on rural Indian reservations. I started getting more and more spasms in my back and neck, along with continued migraines and stress, which made it worse. Eventually I had shooting pain down my right leg constantly from the spasms but continued to work. I didn't want to be a complainer. I began not sleeping as well and had shifts that frequently changed from days to nights, like most doctors do. My immune system was becoming quite weak and I started having more and more pain that I had to work through because there was nobody else to cover my shifts. I wanted so badly to help take care of the underserved populations, but was neglecting myself. I thought I had to and that there was no other choice, that I couldn't change anything in my life and that all of this illness was going to just continue to get worse. I tried a few things like small diet changes and exercise but started feeling like they weren't any use. I rarely saw the sun or got enough sleep. I got strep throat three different times on three different reservations within five months and was treated with three different antibiotic courses. I worked through high fevers with masks on so that I wouldn't have to let any patients be unseen, since in most cases I was the only doctor there. Soon after my third episode of strep throat, I became extremely depressed. I had so much pain physically and emotionally it felt unbearable.

I came back to my home in Arizona and saw my psychiatrist, who had known me for four years by then, through residency and now as a fully-trained doctor.

He had asked on several occasions (as had my prior psychiatrist) if I really thought I was bipolar. At this point I'd even dated a psychiatrist who didn't think I was bipolar. He told me a mix of exhaustion and repeat bacterial infections was depleting my folate, a nutrient that is important for making serotonin, one of the happiness hormones. Without serotonin the antidepressant being used to counteract the depressing features of my mood stabilizer wasn't working. I realized the mood stabilizer also depleted my folate. The two medications were working against each other.

I was quite scared to go off my meds at first, but then after seeing how all the side effects of the initial medications were causing all of my other problems, including my physical problems, I became determined to wean off of them. I started changing my life to be the healthiest possible environment I could be in. I stopped working nights and started working less, getting exercise, improving my diet, and seeing the sunshine. I also started meditating again, only ten minutes a day, and my migraines resolved. I was able to wean off the low dose medications with the close supervision of my psychiatrist. My back pain and spasms also began resolving, along with the shooting pain. It was incredibly painful emotionally because now my brain had to remodel after being changed by medication for so long, but well it was worth it.

I started feeling better and having more energy. I did not know that I would start improving my body so much. It was so much easier to get healthy in my body when I started to believe in myself more. Now I show my patients that they can also take back their health by loving themselves back to better health despite their circumstances.

CHAPTER 3

HOW IT WORKS

"There's more than one way to skin a cat."
– American phrase

W hile I don't want to imagine what it's actually like to skin a cat, the age-old phrase gets to the point of this book—we can accomplish the same thing in many ways. While advertisers would love for us to all think we need the same thing, it's simply not true. There are so many medications that claim to be a one-size-fits-all solution to problems that in actuality may have very different sources. For example, there are many, many causes of depression, from hormones to brain injuries to genetics. Some of these are not necessarily tested for, as there are some things we cannot test for yet; however, time after time patients end up on the same medication that may or may not be useful, since somebody may see a commercial one day describing the symptoms they have and claiming that the "cure" is that particular medication. Some patients will stick with a medication that is causing side effects or not working and continuously raise the dose or try to talk themselves into thinking it's working when it's not. I see this all the time, including in myself. The idea here is to know what will work for you.

Thus, when I give suggestions here in this book, I want you to take them with an understanding that if one thing doesn't work for you then that's fine. Let it go and try another thing. I do suggest though that the other thing you try accomplishes the same goal. For example, if I say, "Eat a leafy green daily" and give a few suggestions, this means eat what works for you. What I don't mean is, "Keep eating a bunch of fast food and no vegetables at all because that's what you're used to and it's too hard to add a vegetable." Some changes will take at least a little bit of effort, but over time will make life much, much simpler. I'm not going to give you a strict diet you need to undertake with every meal planned, because that doesn't work for everybody and is not sustainable. I want people to learn the *principles* here so they can find how they work in their life and then apply them for permanent change. Eventually you will make changes according to what feels right for you instead of what everybody else throws at you. It's extremely freeing.

It might not seem like the small principles in this book will help reverse your disease, but these small steps have consistently proven to make big change with both myself and my patients. "Small things" have been the key to solving big medical mysteries since the beginning of time. Take, for example, hand washing. In 1846, less than two centuries ago, a physician in Vienna noted that women who were delivering in the maternity ward were more likely to get fevers and die when delivered by the physicians than in the midwife clinic. The difference was that physicians would frequently perform autopsies prior to the delivery but not the midwives. The physician then enacted a rule that the physicians must wash hands with chlorine (the best hand cleaner they had at the time) prior to deliveries, and the rates of fever and death plummeted. Even though hand washing seems small, it was literally a matter of life and death before we realized how important it is!

We sometimes assume that because something is small now that it was never a big deal or difficult to change. I'm sure there was plenty of doubt and pushback when hand washing was put into place, just as I'm sure there will be some doubt that the things I suggest in this book will actually help in your life. Just remember there is no such thing as a change too small.

I'm not saying that by the end of the book you will be completely off every medication. The point of this book is to dig up and remodel the foundation that will eventually get you to the point of the least amount of medications. Of course it takes time to reverse disease. However, that disease reversal starts in the mind. After all, there is mounting proof that the mind can start disease in the first place! For example, it's proven that post-traumatic stress disorder (PTSD) creates a change in our DNA called methylation. This means that just experiencing something stressful, without any physical injuries, creates an actual bodily change.[4] Another study that shows that stress reduction can actually improve severe skin diseases like atopic dermatitis, a seriously painful and frustrating chronic disease of the skin that can take many medications and treatments to control over an entire lifetime.[5] The list of diseases linked to stress, such as fibromyalgia, chronic pain, abdominal pain, arthritis, and migraines, is so long that would take many, many books to list and discuss all the studies. At the children's hospital where I did part of my training, there was a full chronic abdominal pain team that was full of—you might have guessed it—therapists and psychiatrists. It is not uncommon to have a child who is brought into the hospital over and over again by an overbearing parent unwilling to accept that the problem may be them and the stress they place on their child. They demand the child undergo hundreds of blood tests and imaging every month that show no physical abnormality to explain the disease; it exposes them to radiation, and worsens the problem. This is because the child is stressed out from the parent and maybe other home factors that are being ignored. As doctors, we have some protocols for things like this that basically include seeing the patient a lot to reassure them—*not* more imaging and tests—and that actually improves the patient. So, basically, stress relief in the form of reassurance to the parent.

Additionally, there is so much proof that the mind controls many diseases in our body. It is proven time and time again that meditation decreases chronic pain. That's right, just calming your mind can in turn calm your body and can decrease the amount of pain you're having. There are studies, too, that the placebo effect has an actual effect. That means that a patient given a fake medication in a study believes that they are getting the real medication and actually improves in the way the medication is supposed to work. The fact that a patient believes they are taking a medication to get better actually improves them. So, couldn't it be true that believing our bodies can take care of their own healing if they have the appropriate materials may actually make us better? If a patient thinks they are going to get better because they are taking a new, fancy medication and gets better in the way they're supposed to get better, that means basically our bodies can usually handle things if we treat them right.

This book is meant to *simplify* your life. Nobody can integrate a thousand new suggestions packed into thirteen chapters into their lives, so I've made a few small lifestyle change suggestions but am mostly leaving it up to you, the reader, to determine what to pursue beyond it. Again, the goal is to make changes that will last for the rest of your life, easily, and to simplify everything. The more research that is uncovered, the more it seems our bodies already know what to do, and there are some traditions that got it right already. The Center for Disease Control gives grants to Native American tribes encouraging us to eat according to the Medicine Wheel, a spiritually-based tradition.[6] This has been shown to decrease diabetes and other inflammatory diseases by giving our bodies what they need. Our bodies can improve by getting back to the basics, rather than by adding more things.

You don't need a medical degree to know that something is not right in your body. However, with the invention of the internet and a million ways to scare ourselves, it is easy to fall down the rabbit hole, destroying our own intuition and turning it into fear because the internet told us we now have something like cancer. Our health can be a terrifying thing if we let it be. It seems every day there is a new disease linked to something we do.

Here I try to explain what is *right* with your health and how to keep doing those good things to have more health. You will gain confidence through seeing all the right that you are doing, not all the problems with you. This leads to making more decisions by listening to yourself and, yes, choosing if you want to go on medications or try something else. Don't discount other forms of improving health, like meditation, as we explore later in the book. However, do not have things done to you that are unproven and may be harmful, like unregulated injections or pills. Even if they are "organic" and "natural" this does not always mean safe if we're given too much or in unconventional ways. For example, when I was in residency there was a patient who died from an IV injection of turmeric. I'm a huge fan of turmeric, but not in experimental ways that are not proven to be safe. The goal by the end of this book is to not need to put much into your body, anyway.

The best way to make permanent change and reverse disease is in the order laid out here in the book, so I will refer to making them that way. You can make the changes in this book out of order if you wish, but you must fully make all of them. Sometimes it's easier to start with some physical actions and then your mind will follow. However, you will not fully reap a permanent change in your life if you don't make each little thing into a lifetime habit in whatever way you can. As they say, it takes twenty-one times in a row to make something into a habit. Start with one thing and do it for twenty-one days, then you will start *wanting* to do it. Eventually your new habit will be integrated into your life and you will feel like something is off if you haven't done it that day. You may also find a way that works better for you, and that is great too. All I ask is that you are fully honest with yourself. Don't fool yourself if you know that something doesn't work for you. Also, don't pretend like you're fully making a change; if *really* you're not, then ask yourself why it's not working. You'll know why it's not working if you're honest. You don't have to tell anybody else if it's embarrassing—though you will find that you start saying the truth because you don't care what people think.

In this book we will first work on acceptance of who you are, then how to know what treatments, if any, are right for you. I know that this may seem like a strange place to start, but I have noticed that it is not until somebody is accepting of themselves that they believe in their ability to change. If you aren't, you'll find yourself making some changes temporarily until your willpower runs out, and then ending up back at square one. If you keep the same core beliefs you've always had, then any outer, physical change will not be sustained. Just like a house with a cracked foundation, until the foundation is excavated and replaced a new building cannot be built. This is the same as your beliefs and habits—without new beliefs your habits will revert back, which is why the first habit change I suggest is changing those beliefs. Since if you do something twenty-one days in a row it becomes a habit, I would suggest you try each thing for thirty days with *real* effort before deciding it doesn't work for you. The initial suggestions of creating self-confidence and gratitude are not just made up out of nowhere. They are the most important part of sustaining self-sufficiency after making changes. There are studies supporting them in the chapters that follow, but the most important evidence you will find is your own change. For the sake of this book, you have to do something thirty times to feel the change for yourself.

I will progress then into some very simple practical tips about diet and exercise—again, with what I have found in both studies and personal experience. These may be the same suggestions you have had in the past that seemed too simple, but they are the easiest starting point I have found. Once you've mastered these simple things you will get a good grasp on what kinds of goals to set for yourself that you can accomplish. Then you will be ready to accomplish whatever you want, knowing you can do it one step at a time.

Please, please do not just stop your medications cold turkey; this is dangerous for almost any medication and could even lead to death. I'll say it again: *Please, please do not just stop your medications cold turkey; this is dangerous for almost any medication and could even lead to death.* Once you have laid the groundwork of changing your core beliefs and have taken ample time to think about it, discuss tapering down with the prescriber of the medication to do so safely.

Above all, make sure you find all that's right with you. The more you continue to find the right, the wrong just seems to fall away. Eventually whatever you feel is wrong with you won't take up your time or energy because you're so focused on what's right. This is also true of diseases, I have found. As the wallpaper on my phone reminds me, *"Be gentle with yourself. You're doing the best you can."*

CHAPTER 4

BEING WRONG IS RIGHT!

"You can't think your way into right action, but you can act your way into right thinking."
– Bill Wilson

As I surveyed people during the writing of this book, I confirmed that most people have felt the way I felt at one time—alone and overwhelmed. People try to claim it's human nature, that we are all supposed to be in competition and there is a limited amount of success we are all fighting for. They start to believe that in order to be happy we need to have more, be more, do more. The phrase "has nothing to show for it" commonly refers to material goods, but what if we stop and change what success means? I have found it to be way more true that "money can't buy happiness"—and also that things to do not equal happiness. There are studies that show that winning the lottery does not make happiness, but in many cases created a depressive episode.[7] In the *Forbes* yearly "happiest places on earth" articles, they repeatedly state that the happiest places are full of people who feel connected to others, especially when times are tough.[8] You may believe that "survival of the fittest" is part of our evolution and that that's what Darwin wrote in his book *The Descent of Man*, where the phrase "survival of the fittest" came from. Actually though, he only writes twice about "survival of the fittest" and mentions love ninety-five times. According to The Darwin Project, "he writes of selfishness twelve times but ninety-two times of moral sensitivity, of competition nine times but twenty-four times of mutuality and mutual aid."[9]

One study observes players of a game that includes partners. In the game if you decide to go against your partner during a round you will gain immediate rewards, though if you cooperate you will later get greater rewards together; however, your partner can still decide not to cooperate later and you will not get anything. They found that an area of the brain that is activated with reward, the ventral striatum, is activated when a player cooperates *even when the partner does not cooperate.* They also found that a player's ventral striatum is less active when they choose not to cooperate *despite immediately getting a material reward.* What this means is our area of reward is more activated with cooperation than any material gain.[10]

I talked a lot in the last chapter about how it's important to focus on how much of us is right. This should start with cooperation as it makes us automatically feel rewarded, whether or not the other person gives back. Hence "act your way into better thinking" is more of a reality than just a fun catch phrase. Remember how good it felt when you went out of your way to do a kind deed for somebody despite not receiving any physical reward? That's not because we just imagined it felt good—our brains were actually activated! How much depression would be resolved if we all went around cooperating?

Clearly our bodies wouldn't naturally activate the reward area when we worked together if it wasn't our human nature. I don't know how the population went so awry with these "facts" about how it's a "cold hard world and you have to shoulder the burden on your own." I do know I also believed it and had my own depression leading to physical ailments that resolved when I changed my actions into cooperation. This meant I had to break down my own walls of always having to be right. This listening and admitting that maybe we don't know things is a vulnerable state because the popular opinion seems to be that this is not how we should be—but that is just not true.

We have to change what it *means* to be wrong to knowing that if we don't know something we aren't "dumb" or "stupid" as a person, but rather learning just like everybody else. What I believe, and teach my daughter, is that the only time we are doing something wrong is if we are knowingly hurting another living thing, either physically or emotionally, and continue to do so. If somebody alerts us to how we are hurting somebody or something else that we were unaware of prior to this, we change it. However, if somebody accuses us of being at fault because they are unable to see their part in things, we don't need to absorb their opinion and change to suit them. Trying to be what everybody else wants us to be is stressful, exhausting, and detrimental to our health. People talk about how we aren't perfect, but I disagree. We *are* perfect exactly as we are. If you don't think it's true, then re-evaluate what your definition of perfect is. I am one hundred percent always perfectly me. *Nobody* is as perfect at being me as I am. I don't always love everything about myself, but know that I can examine and change or learn to accept it all. We learn a definition of perfect from the expectations others place on us and then uncomfortably try to be something we aren't. I remember feeling particularly anxious about not being a "perfect" doctor and my stepmother saying to me, "It must be hard because you were already such a perfectionist" without any mention of how my home environment could have shaped it. I don't think we are born trying to fit into what somebody else thinks we should do. You don't see toddlers trying to be like somebody else until they are conditioned to behave however their environment teaches them.

I truly believe we miss out on a lot in our life because we are taught we are somehow supposed to know everything all the time. We get in our heads that if we don't know everything all the time, something is somehow fundamentally flawed with us. We are taught to "fake it till you make it," meaning act confident even if you don't know what you're doing, until you do know. But if we did know everything all the time then we would have nothing to learn. If there was one universal truth, then we would all think the same and never have disagreements. Also, if you really step back and let go of what it might *mean* about you to be wrong, you might realize of course we don't all know everything all the time. It's even silly to imagine it! I may be a doctor, but that doesn't mean I somehow know more about everything. I still have to call somebody else to fix the electricity or the plumbing. Thank goodness there are many people with different knowledge areas, or we would all have the same job! Again, this reiterates that we *need* cooperation and appreciation of all.

I think it would be pretty boring if we all knew everything all the time because then we would never make any new discoveries. I would not get to see different art, taste different foods, or even be pleasantly surprised! There would never be an opportunity to hear different opinions and analyze what I think about something. I find that the more I know, the more there is to know. Obviously if I beat myself up for all, or any, of the things I don't know, I could be endlessly criticizing myself. If I felt bad for not knowing how to wire a house, then maybe I would be too embarrassed to ask an electrician to come do it for me. I could try to fool myself into thinking that I knew best how to do it, then do something wrong and never have electricity. Then, because I didn't want to admit I didn't know something, I would sit around with no electricity in my house and pretend I was happy without electricity, all because I was afraid of saying, "I don't know how to do this."

I know that seems like a funny and extreme example, but there are things happening like this all the time, both in and out of medicine. People can be fantastic at pretending like they know what they are talking about and maybe even believe that they do, in fact, know it. However, the way they know how to do something from their experience is not always the best way for us. The key here is to listen to what somebody has to say and try to understand it from their viewpoint, then decide if that applies to you. Truly listening means that you don't jump to defend why you thought what you thought or justify why you didn't know. You just sit, listen, let it all sink in, and thank others for their advice. Afterward you have learned something that, even if it's just opinion, may improve your life. When you truly listen to understand another person without defending yourself, you are creating cooperation and decreasing long-term stress. This can apply from doctors to friends and even children. You don't have to do what everybody says, but respect the human in front of you doing their best to help. Stress is the root of most diseases, or at least plays a part, even if the disease is part genetic. It is also the root of the bad habits we "can't change no matter what" that create disease, like smoking, eating, drinking, gambling. Less stress and more cooperation overall will eventually create more happiness in general and less need to fill ourselves impulsively with things that are hurting us.

Before I continue, please let me clear up a common misconception. Doctors *do not get kickbacks for prescribing certain medications.* This is so illegal it is, in fact, a felony for them to do so. We aren't "pill pushing" because we get paid, and if you suspect your doctor is, please ask them about it before making frivolous claims. Society has created this big divide between Western medicine and other forms of healing. I grew up in a family that was very heavily Western medicine-oriented, and so I never learned what things like natural herbs or essential oils could do for my body. As a matter of fact, I spent most of my life up until very recently completely believing that there was nothing better than or equal to Western medicine, because that's what I was surrounded by, people who believed the same thing.

There are so many forms of "medicine" patients have missed out on because of our inability to admit our way is not always best. For example, I use turmeric myself every morning, and it seems to help with stress and feeling down or overwhelmed and ultimately helps me keep things like migraines and chronic pain in check without all the side effects. Additionally, when I lived in Arizona I personally knew somebody who was hired by the Mayo Clinic to do Reiki on the patients admitted there, as it seemed to benefit patients. I know another person who does some work at a military hospital that used to be thought of as "energy healing" but actually benefits soldiers with PTSD so much that it's scientifically proven to help—without any extra medications. Some physicians and patients don't want to think that there are things as good for you, or better for you, as Western medicine because that's what we've learned.

This makes sense based on our environment and training. I will talk about being a Western medicine physician here, but see if you can relate it to your job. Doctors of Western medicine spend years of their lives training. Medical school is so intensive that it seems that there is no way you could put any more classes in than there already are. We literally lose our social lives and happiness believing we are going to help others. Unfortunately, we are unable to fit in classes on things like acupuncture, homeopathy, or naturopathy. I don't know that medical schools teach that these things are wrong or do not work, we just don't have the time to also fit that in. However, we do teach doctors that the medicine we know is the best possible based on current evidence. There is evidence to support some things that are not Western medicine but, again, there isn't time to teach *all* of it.

Doctors memorize hundreds of medications, their common side effects, who to use them for, who not to use them with, what situation to use them in, what they might interact with, what time of day to take them, what to take them with, and what not to take them with. As you can imagine, just the medicines are overwhelming and no one doctor can know everything about all of them. However, doctors must believe and are taught that this is the best solution we have. I say they must believe it because if you don't believe something is going to work, then why would you use it when it can literally mean life or death for you and your patient? This is assuming each doctor would use the same treatments on their patients that they would use on themselves. I don't personally know of any doctor who is genuinely hoping to harm their patients. I am speaking about the majority of doctors who started studying medicine believing it is the best way to help others. Those who were, like me, taught that becoming a doctor was the ultimate in helping others and didn't even know that things like naturopathy exist. As you might imagine, if a doctor does not even know about other treatments but has literally dedicated their life to knowing Western medicine, then it would be difficult for them to learn that there are a lot of options just as good, if not better. This goes for other things, like surgeries or other procedures, too. The best surgeons I know are those who were willing to try almost everything else before a surgery instead of jumping right to it because they understood all of the risks of long-term complications to patients.

People will roll their eyes and say, "doctors think they are God." Sure, there are people of every profession who think they are perfect; however, I think more frequently than not it is the patient who tells a doctor they should be perfect. Although in theory most people know their doctor is also a human doing their best, there are times this feels forgotten. I've heard people ask me so many times if they should sue their doctors for using a treatment that was standard of care (meaning the best treatment known in medicine at the time) because they didn't like the side effect. For example, one patient had his heart suddenly stop one day at the gym, but was revived with CPR. After the open heart surgery that ultimately saved his life, he asked if he should sue those who did the CPR for breaking his ribs. I was shocked. He was alive and doing very well and wanted money from the other human being that did their best. This story is not that unique, either. I have both heard similar horror stories and been threatened for similar situations. Doctors are *not* God; we cannot magically cure you without any side effects. We become terrified of lack of perfection and hence can over-treat or over-refer because of constant threat of being sued or reported for fully appropriate medical care (and in most cases, above and beyond care).

This is a problem that ultimately leads to patients hurt from the over-treatment. Obviously I don't think a doctor who is making horrendous mistakes repeatedly and refuses to learn or fix them should continue to practice medicine, but at what point are other people going to let doctors also be human? At what point will patients know that when they come to see the doctor we are also doing our best and fully support you if you want a second opinion? It should never a problem for a patient to just genuinely want to get another opinion from somebody with a different viewpoint.

I will perform a full workup of what could be causing a patient's symptoms to be sure that it is not something that requires intervention first. Unfortunately, we are paid by insurance companies based on making every patient *happy, not necessarily healthy.* This has been proven to create worse outcomes, yet insurances will base whether or not doctors get reimbursed for their work based on patient satisfaction, *not* health. One study even shows higher mortality rates with greater survey-based satisfaction.[11] You may have seen surveys in the mail about your hospital or doctor visit. It is statistically less likely that you will fill them out if you were happy with your visit, but guess who *does* fill them out? Mostly people who are unhappy. When doctors bill insurance companies, they get reimbursed based on patient satisfaction. I'm not talking about getting all the money they bill for, either—I mean *maybe* a quarter of it. On a scale from one to ten, the answer has to be a ten for it to "count" as the patient being satisfied. I'm not talking about millions of dollars we can do without, either; I'm talking about enough money to pay for all of the expenses of running a business and paying for our basic life expenditures. Primary care doctors go bankrupt and quit medicine all the time because in order to be reimbursed enough they have to see a patient about every fifteen to twenty minutes in an eight-hour day and be on the computer documenting double that amount of time. So, if I actually spend ten minutes with twenty-four patients in a day, that's only four hours; however, you can count on an average of about three times that amount of time, so twelve hours, following up labs, documenting, calling, refilling prescriptions, and various other tasks. So our "eight-hour day" quickly becomes twelve hours, even when we don't get to spend as much time with our patients as we want.

Most doctors I know, including myself, also hate not having time to listen to and interact with their patients. We want to also know them and create a trusting relationship. We want to do the best possible thing for each patient and hear their whole story. Hopefully by now you see what kind of environment this creates. A world where a patient demands things that may not be necessary and may even be detrimental to the patient's health because, if not, the doctor may not be able to practice medicine. The notoriously low pay for primary care doctors is leading to an ever-increasing number of medical students choosing higher-paying fields.

Let me reiterate that you are absolutely allowed to have genuine concern about your care, express those concerns, and have all your questions answered. I believe patients should be given every option a doctor knows of and decisions should be made together if it is appropriate. You never *have* to do just what a doctor says and you are absolutely allowed to ask questions. If they don't want to answer them then you are fully allowed to talk to somebody else, but may have to find them yourself. However, in the ER I'm not going to wait for a patient who is unconscious to wake up after a severe car accident before performing the procedure that may save their life.

Be careful in pointing fingers though. Although it is well known that medical errors can cause death, natural medicine can also cause death. Because supplements are not regulated, they are not studied as much as Western medications. I myself see an alternative medicine practitioner in conjunction with my primary care doctor, and we integrate both based on what works best for me. However, I have treated many patients in the hospital who have died from over-utilization of these alternatives. For example, I once saw a nine-year-old who died of liver failure from supplements prescribed by an alternative medicine practitioner. I have personally treated patients who have died from damage to the arteries in their necks from chiropractors. The overwhelming issue with all of this is that there was a lack of moderation (something that most people don't do well, including all forms of medicine, because we don't realize we are over-doing it most times). As a society we are taught "if some is good, more must be better" and neither Western nor alternative medicine are any exception. I don't tell you all of this so that you will dislike practitioners of alternative medicine; as I stated above, I myself see one in addition to my primary care doctor. I tell you this because assuming that one thing is all perfect while the other thing is all bad is a problem.

The idea is moderation and acceptance that what works best for somebody else may not be ultimately what works best for you. Try adding or subtracting *one* thing at a time unless something has already been proven to not be effective. There are some protocols in which the evidence is well-studied that I must prescribe more than one antibiotic for a period of time or the infection will not improve. I'm not a big fan of doing so, but it's proven that the double antibiotic works and the single does not. You can then ask your doctor what would help with side effects, and if they don't know then you can ask a naturopath and vice versa. Then bring what you're doing to the practitioner (whether alternative or Western) so they can integrate and maybe use it to help future patients. Here is a part of cooperation I wish more Western *and* alternative medicine practitioners and patients would get on board with. Stop writing off the other fully, learn what you can, and integrate what works for you.

Who I think are the best practitioners of Western or alternative medicine are those who see the place for everything. I chose my primary care physician based on his willingness to integrate other things into my Western medicine treatment, just as I chose my alternative medicine practitioners based on their willingness to work with what Western medicine I choose to integrate into my alternative healing. Several alternative medicine practitioners have said to me, "If I have to go to the emergency room for a life-threatening illness or to have emergency surgery and I have to choose, I would absolutely choose Western medicine. If it comes to primary care, then I prefer more natural." I feel that this is the best approach, to be able to see a time and place for things. Which gets us back to cooperation being the best for everybody involved.

The first step in this book to reversing your disease is to start cooperating with others. Do as many random acts of kindness without receiving any reward or telling anybody about it as you can, like a kindness superhero. Also, it is found that happiness comes from gratitude, not the other way around. It is therefore imperative you start writing a list of ten new things you're grateful for every morning. Remember, do it thirty days in a row before you decide it works or does not work for you, *and actually write it down.* You must take action and your mind will follow.

CHAPTER 5

APPRECIATE YOURSELF

"To enjoy good health, to bring true happiness to one's family, to bring peace to all, one must first discipline and control one's own mind. If a man can control his mind he can find the way to Enlightenment, and all wisdom and virtue will naturally come to him."

– The Buddha

I t is interesting to me how much we discount the mind-body connection for most of the population. I find that patients easily talk about their physical disease or pain, but emotional pain seems to be off limits. It is strange to me that somehow talking about cancer elicits sympathy, but depression inspires a judgment of character. I believe this is because the population does not understand that most disease starts as something emotional. There are so many books written by people who thoroughly researched the mind-body connection. This struck me during my residency, when I saw a patient who did exactly this. Let's call her Jane. Jane came to see me because her usual primary care doctor was not available. In a resident clinic, patients frequently saw a different doctors because residents would have varying availability. Jane came in for an evaluation of her healed wound. She told me that she had been bitten by a dog eight months prior and wanted me to take a look at the healing wound, which was about two inches long. It looked like it was well-healed and I reassured her. She then sheepishly brought up, "At night when I hear dogs barking I wake up and I'm so scared, I can hardly sleep." I then realized, this is actually what she's here for. I was about to explain to her that this was completely normal. Before I could start talking, she tried to justify what she was feeling because of embarrassment. She went on to say, "I know this is really stupid and weak and I shouldn't feel this way." I looked Jane in the eyes and said, "What you are feeling is very real and it's okay.

Nothing is wrong with you for being scared." Jane then burst into tears. She expressed that nobody before me had told her it was okay to be scared. That fear is a normal response. I was stunned; surely there had been somebody in her family or a friend who had expressed understanding about fear from an event. Jane was so scared she was not sleeping, which was going to create a *lot* more problems if she hadn't had the opportunity to discuss why she was stressed with somebody who was understanding.

Stress leading to lack of sleep can raise things like cortisol levels and blood sugar (among other things), which over time wreak havoc on your body.[12] These seemingly-little events can cause trauma in different people. If we try to ignore the emotional distress, we are letting our body stay inflamed and our "fight-or-flight" (sympathetic nervous system) response is staying on constantly. Part of what this overworking of our sympathetic nervous system means is that your body puts priority on the function of organs you need when you're trying to do something like run from a tiger. So it makes sense that the blood would go to your eyes, to your heart, to your mind, and not to things like your digestive system. This leads to something that is so common but we are embarrassed to talked about: chronic constipation. While there can be many, many physical manifestations of stress, constipation is a frequently underestimated and therefore undertreated issue. This chronic constipation can cause weight gain and lead to issues like depression, headaches, and fatigue. Then we come back to the doctor wondering why we're chronically constipated, ignoring that it may be because we are still stressed out from something and nothing is actually wrong with our bodies because our bodies are appropriately responding to what we still see as a threat.

Nothing is wrong with you for seeing something scary as a threat. As a matter of fact, research has shown that our DNA actually changes from seeing—just seeing—something stressful. Research has found that PTSD in soldiers causes methylation of DNA. That means the stress of seeing combat causes a literal change in DNA. This likely applies to most types of non-physical trauma. This has been proven over and over in other populations, including mice. This isn't some unconfirmed new age idea. Now the research is focusing on how to undo it. One of my favorite methods, shown to be promising in mice, is having a "a low-stress and enriched environment in adult life."[13] Some of us laugh—there's no way with our world that we could have a low-stress adulthood. I agree; if you believe that life should be a certain way and if it's not that way, then it's stressful. For example, if you believe that you will never have to sit in traffic and then you do every day, of course it stresses you out. If you change your mind into thinking, "Yeah, traffic is a part of life," then you find ways to make it enjoyable and it doesn't stress you out.

What another study has shown is that you can decrease these kinds of health problems by changing what you perceive as stressful. This is not some Yogi, monk, meditation guru idea. You don't have to meditate eight hours a day to think things that were previously stressful are not stressful. Look around you. Think of the things other people think are extremely stressful that you do not in fact find stressful. For example, divorce. I have been divorced. It can be extremely difficult and I don't think anybody should try to pretend that it's easy and fun, but through some self-love practices (one of which is the next step to creating reversal of disease that I will discuss at the end of the chapter), we can learn to be gentle with ourselves. We can change the idea that divorce was never supposed to happen to us and now that it has we are bad people. The divorce rate is about fifty percent or higher; why wouldn't it be me who got divorced? Then I go on to be gentle with myself. I stopped thinking I'm the only one in the world who has ever experienced this, because I'm not. And even though the details of why or how it happened may be much different than other people's, there will almost always be other people who have been through something similar. I think the key is to find other people who understand and can normalize it. If you're around people who constantly tell you not to feel, and you're pushing your emotions down, then guess what? Those feelings are still there, causing your body to respond appropriately—meaning, your body is responding as if a tiger is constantly threatening it. So tell your body, "Great job and thank you, but now let's give it a rest and understand this can be normal," and start moving forward. However, be careful in finding people to relate to (like others who have been divorced, for example) who continually speak negatively about it for years and years without trying to improve or change. Watch out that you are not blaming your lack of happiness on somebody or something else.

When I had difficult times in life, my family seemed to separate themselves from me because feelings were uncomfortable. I don't think they're very abnormal in that. People get so uncomfortable when we express real feelings, and they think that we are weird or sometimes abnormal. The more I have observed people as a physician, the more I realize the abnormal people are those who think feelings are weird. The really abnormal thing is to suppress emotion. Look at a child. They don't sit around and wonder who's going to think what if they cry—oh, and guess what? They cry, let it all out, and then go about their day. They're much happier and they don't hold in these grudges and anger forever. I'm talking about the little kid on the playground who gets mad because another child hit them. The other child was probably doing something based on their instincts that they were threatened. Both children will cry and go see their adult who comforts them, and then they come back and one apologizes to the other, and the kids let it go, way better than parents, usually. Ten years from then, they don't still have a grudge and anger toward the little kid that hit them. They don't even have a grudge the next day! They'll let go, forgive, move on.

I'm not suggesting that if somebody's hitting you in an abusive sense that you just let it go and move on and keep letting them do that. Absolutely not—get somewhere safe. I'm saying it's okay to cry, it's okay to run around, it's okay to throw a toddler-like tantrum on the floor. Maybe not in public yet…until the rest of humanity comes around to the idea, at least. Where and when did we start believing that these absolutely normal responses to things were not normal? If we weren't supposed to cry then why would everybody have that capacity? Why would it happen naturally and then we push it back down? It's not like we all stand there willingly trying to start crying, then push it down. As a baby we all have newborn reflexes. Crying is one of them. It's like we allow our bodies to do things like breathe, but not some other normal physiologic responses like crying. Crying can be a wonderful way our bodies naturally let go of these feelings.

When I was in medical school, a newly-single mom mid-divorce who was doing everything I could to stay on track in school, I was given what is probably one of my favorite compliments. My friend told me, "It's a good thing you can laugh at things, because if you couldn't you would be screwed." I definitely could have taken this as an insult, but realized he was right. There absolutely are times when I'm not finding humor in something. But if you can really step back and see the irony in some of the situations we're in, then they become hilarious. Here's an example from that time. I had been married and divorced, had a child, and started medical school before the age of twenty-three. You know how many people insulted me, both to my face and behind my back, who really knew very little about the situation? Many, many people. You know what I told them? "I'm front-loading my life so that I'll be free to do whatever I want later." I said it and *actually believed it was funny.* It wasn't my first instinct—I felt bad at first—but I couldn't change it so I learned to find humor. If I can find some humor in all of that just by changing my thoughts about it, I think anybody can. Do things become easier because all of a sudden life doesn't throw curveballs? No. They become easier because you realize you're not in charge of that and you can laugh knowing that you're not alone in this. This is how I think an adult can have what seems to be a "a low-stress and enriched environment in adult life," which is showing promising research to reverse the damage done to our DNA from PTSD, as mentioned above. See how I'm saying our perception of things can literally hurt or heal our own bodies?

If you think to yourself, "I can never be stress-free or perceive things like that because that would mean I don't care or want to get better," I have news for you. I, too, have felt that way. I thought that I was the only person who had been diagnosed as bipolar. You can imagine how I would never, ever want to tell anybody about this. For years I was ashamed and the people around me used those things to shame me and not take responsibility for their own actions. It was an endless cycle. Eventually, with about ten minutes or less of meditation a day, I started realizing I didn't express the symptoms that we will work on in another chapter. In time, I overturned the diagnosis with the appropriate help and guidance from my doctor and therapist. We understood together how my body was appropriately responding to the situations around me. How there was good reason for me to try to find things to dampen or suppress my fight-or-flight response. Why I wasn't sleeping. When I got the proper support and learned all of the good about me, despite what I thought were lifelong, chronic diseases, they resolved. This means I didn't necessarily need all the Western medicine or anything else I may have done to feel better. This also applies to my physical chronic illnesses, like severe migraines. They didn't start until well into adulthood. Yet there was nothing to explain why I had them. I was taking multiple medications a day to try to control them. I was even having Botox injected into the back of my head to relax the muscles so I wasn't getting them all the time. Over time and as I worked on appreciating myself, I needed the medications less and eventually the migraines also went away. I have seen this in patients with diabetes, high blood pressure, fibromyalgia, almost anything that you can think of that doesn't involve something we are born without or with. I think there's a lot to explore even with inborn issues, but that is a much deeper topic for another book.

One example I like to give here about how we can view even our physical illnesses is from my own experience. I was born with a hole between the top two chambers of my heart. I found this out around the age of twenty-four, after my father had a mini stroke from his own hole between the top two chambers of his heart. I could sit around and be sad that I was born with this; however, it was easily fixed with a closure device that they put in by going through one of my veins. And I have not had a problem with it since. I could certainly use this heart defect as an excuse to avoid things like exercising, but I don't. I do have to have more check-ups for the rest of my life and did have to take medications for the condition for a while— more things I could use as a crutch or constantly worry about. Occasionally I have some funny heart rhythms, which can be a little bit scary but resolve on their own—and I could also choose to sit around and be afraid that one day they don't resolve on their own. I choose instead to let it go and deal with something like that if it even occurs. The worry of it would probably create more heart palpitations anyway! Instead, I think of how grateful I am that I didn't have any of the severe complications from this. For example, during pregnancy women with this particular hole in their heart can have severe strokes. As a matter of fact, they are thirty times more likely to have a stroke. When I was pregnant, I did not know I had the heart condition. I remember doing an OB/GYN rotation in medical school shortly after discovering the hole in my heart. We went to see a patient who was five months pregnant, twenty-one years old, who had had a severe stroke leaving the left side of her body paralyzed. I'm so grateful that I did not, but feel that having a near miss has made me more compassionate to patients who weren't as lucky, and not just with heart-related conditions. I'm not saying you should feel bad if you're the person who did have the complications, but I'm saying usually there's something way worse that could have happened. I could have had severe heart problems I was born with that required many, many open heart surgeries—even some as an adult. I know a doctor born with severe heart issues like this. He doesn't sit around and think about it all the time and limit what he can and can't do because of it. He takes an opportunity to look at all the things he *does* have. He became a doctor, his brain works well, and he appreciates all that is right about himself. If you focus on the things that are going wrong, you're going to find them. However, that not only hurts your self-esteem and causes stress, but continues to hurt your body more and more—like changing your DNA, as above.

The small but very easy new habit we are working on here is this: what's right with you? Every day, write down five things that are right with you. For me it might look like this:

- My heart works well with just a small device
- I gave up my seat without thinking about it in the waiting room
- I had six carrots today

- I went on a brisk ten-minute walk instead of continuing to sit all day
- I smiled at somebody who was not smiling

This may sound too simple, but this is another step in reversing disease. At the beginning of this chapter I gave examples of chronic physical problems that can come about from emotional distress, then spoke about how low stress can reverse these, but not in the way you might think of "low stress," but rather stress reduction by changing what we think of as stressful and not stressful by changing our perception. The exercise above is the way we change our minds into looking for good. Like the last chapter where we started making gratitude lists, *writing down* what is right with us as an action changes our minds into starting to look for what is right. I probably don't have to remind you, but will anyway, to do this for at least thirty days in a row before deciding if it works for you or not. Have fun with it too! Laugh at yourself! You can absolutely change how you perceive things; it's much easier than you think.

CHAPTER 6

TAKE RESPONSIBILITY
FOR YOUR HEALTH

"No one can make you feel inferior without your consent."

– Eleanor Roosevelt

I remember the first time I shadowed a doctor to start exploring what specialty I might be interested in. I was in college and she was a gynecologist, let's call her Dr. Jones. We were in clinic seeing the very first patient of the day and Dr. Jones was describing to the patient the options for the illness she was there for. The first option was lifestyle changes and the second was medication. Of course the patient could absolutely do both or neither, as was discussed with her as well. Medication side effects were thoroughly discussed, as was what she would need to do in order to just reverse it all on her own. Dr. Jones asked if the patient had any questions, and she said no. Then an awkward silence ensued for about thirty seconds, after which Dr. Jones asked what the patient decided. Again, another weird silence ensued. Dr. Jones told the patient she would step out for five minutes and then come back to decide and discuss. We stepped out and saw another patient, then came back. The patient said she would like the medication, as exercising would be too much work. Dr. Jones was happy to provide her with the medication they had decided on. After we walked out the door, I felt confused about what all the uncomfortable silence was about. Without me having to ask, Dr. Jones turned to me and said, "You know all that weird silence? That's because the patient is waiting for some magical option that requires no work and fixes everything without side effects." Then I understood what was going on, not because that patient had unreasonable expectations...because *all* of us have unreasonable expectations. Even doctors.

Everywhere you turn, there are buzzwords flying around like "miracle pill," "unbelievable results," "magic secret," The list goes on. I'm here to tell you that there's no such thing. Does that mean getting better has to be hard and take years to improve? Also no. What I have found is that if anything or anybody claims to have something that magically cures a problem a lot of people have, then they are lying or just haven't discovered its issues. Remember Fen-Phen? It seemed like a magic bullet for weight loss until people were having heart attacks and dying. There are so many other examples that describing them would take too many books that my editor has not yet been paid to edit, so I'll let you do your own research if you're interested in them. The point is, don't wait until somebody else comes up with some magic thing. They won't. I have said this many times to many patients *including myself—Nobody else will put your health first.* Let it sink in while I repeat it—*Nobody else will put your health first.* Not your spouse, your parents, your children, or your doctor. Not because we don't care, but because we have our own world, including health, to manage, too.

That being said, we still like to be mad at people for not acting how we want them to act. Sometimes justifiably, too. How could I not be mad at the person that attempted to rape me? I think it is very justified for me to be angry and scared about that. Then I believe I am justified in being angry at the lack of support from my family, who couldn't even talk about it because they were uncomfortable. Then I could start to feel ashamed of how I'm making somebody else uncomfortable about the attempted rape just by talking about it. Now I don't want to talk about it, because I've been taught it makes others uncomfortable—and what is wrong with me for doing that? Now I'm stressed out because I'm pushing down my traumatic experience. This revs up my sympathetic nervous system (that fight-or-flight reflex in the previous chapter). I sleep less now, even though there's no current threat, then cortisol (a stress hormone we discussed in the previous chapter) is released, then my blood sugar is chronically elevated, then I gain weight, and then comes diabetes, heart disease, etc. It gets worse, too, and then I have even more sleep issues, I'm more stressed out, the cortisol is released more.... See how being mad at another person gets out of control and begins affecting my health?

Yes, there are reasons to get justifiably angry, but when it's hurting you then you're giving them your health. I absolutely endorse speaking up to the proper mental health professional when something terrible happens. If you need to be on a medication for a while because you or somebody else's safety is at risk, that's also okay. Accept what's going to work for you. I also believe you shouldn't *pretend* you don't care when you do. If you have to find the right audience to vent about something happening initially until it's all out, then do it! For me, that usually means a therapist because sometimes talking to people around me doesn't quite do the trick. If I feel like I can't fully talk about everything without judgment, I'm not excavating it all. When we have received validation for our anger and pain, there is a point when we finally get to choose that it's just hurting us now. It's different for everybody and every event, so be gentle with yourself in fully letting it all out. Eventually there is a change that happens that only you know, so pay attention. The change is that you stop needing to process and it's time to let go.

There is a fantastic book called *The Language of Emotions* by Karla McLaren that, along with my therapist, helped me clarify how I knew I had processed it and that holding onto it was hurting me now. In this book she helps by taking the reader through exercises that help identify an emotion by how it feels physically so we can disconnect from judgment of the emotion. For example, if I feel "a lump in my throat" instead of "sadness," it's easier for me to disconnect and therefore not push away or try to suppress the sadness. She then does a beautiful job of putting into context that our emotions are not wrong but are telling us something. For example, she speaks about anger, something I felt ashamed about having for most of my life. However, as I grew older I learned my other siblings, who had been in the same situation as me growing up, had the same feelings. Through my therapist, I learned to say thank you to my anger for telling me somebody had crossed a boundary, then identifying what it was, and speaking my truth. Then I let it go without having to control the other person or hide from the anger. In the past I may have just pushed it all the way down until it came back up as rage.

The other aspect is not to blindly trust every therapist to tell you when you "should be done." You will need to start trusting yourself. After I felt unafraid of my feelings and just felt them on my own without justifying, I was able to let go. That is when I knew continuing to be mad was hurting my health. Don't try to suppress or change those feelings because you think they should be a different way. Your body processes feelings as bodily sensations beautifully if you just let it.

Here are the best ways I have found to let go of things. This is the order I do them in, but you can certainly do it another way if it works for you.

1. First, write a letter you won't send—and don't hold back. Write everything you are mad or happy about. Write about the things you miss or what pains you. Again, this isn't going to be sent, so no reason not to write everything.

Then, write a letter from the person you're writing to, as if you told them all this and they saw it your way and said exactly what you wish they would say. Third, write back to them as if you had gotten a sincere apology and tell them thank you and what boundaries you'll put in the relationship/how the relationship should be going forward. Sometimes that means "I hope to never see you again" and that's also okay. Then you can burn the letters (safely) or get rid of them permanently somehow. You don't need your processing to be accidentally found by somebody else after you've let it go!

2. Pretend like you are the publicist for the person who wronged you and you can't lie. So, pretend like it is literally your job to make them look good and you have to find as many good things about them as possible that are true. This is particularly good for people who are going to remain in your life, who you still have to see. As I said, think of things that are true. If you think there aren't any, then you aren't trying hard enough.

3. Remember a time that you did something similar or close to what the other person did. Are you mad that your friend continually blows you off? If you're honest with yourself,

you have done the same to somebody else. Remember that time.

4. Ho'oponopono. A Hawaiian Forgiveness Ritual. Why does this work? I don't know or pretend to know, but I do it when nothing else works. You can find easy instructions on the internet. I use the short book *Ho'oponopono: The Hawaiian Forgiveness Ritual as the Key to Your Life's Fulfillment* by Ulrich E. Dupree.

There are a million ways to let go of things, so find a way that works for you. You are literally handing over your health to somebody who has done something "wrong" to you. They are human too. We have all made mistakes. Those who can't see where they were wrong have the most pain inside. That doesn't mean you need to try to fix them at the risk of your health. Forgive and let go without taking on their issues that affect your health.

If you're living in close quarters with somebody who you are always having a strong emotional response to, then don't kid yourself into thinking you are somehow separate. There is research that shows that if we analyze EKGs (those little squiggles we do in the emergency room and office for your heart) then we can detect how somebody is feeling, between anger and appreciation.[14] Additionally, there is preliminary research showing that a person can coordinate their brainwaves (via EEG) to another person's heartbeat (EKG).[15] The researchers state that they aren't sure what exactly this means about how much detection of the heartbeat has an effect on our feelings and physical body. However, if we can record my brain coordinating with somebody's heartbeat that is within eighteen inches of me, then I wouldn't be surprised if it has some sort of effect we just can't measure yet. So, if I we can detect what emotion somebody is having from their EKG, and our brains can coordinate with somebody else's heart, perhaps we are taking on their emotions, whether they tell us or not. Perhaps we are fooling ourselves if we think we aren't affected by our friend/coworker/spouse's negativity. There is something you can do about it, though. If you can detect them, maybe they can detect you too, and changing your attitude about them will change theirs about you.

Maybe you are actually the initial instigator of the anger and grouchiness by holding in anger that was undealt with. Just because somebody doesn't yell doesn't mean their internal anger is not felt by others. I know when I am around somebody who seems very grouchy and isn't usually, I have to own my side. Perhaps what I'm holding in is affecting the other person through the path I just mentioned. Maybe they are irritated because I am really angry with them and they are "detecting" it. There is definitely more research to be done because we don't know for sure. However, don't just assume that somebody else is being mean and you are a completely innocent bystander who did nothing. First, we change how we feel about the other person as above and let go; then, without having to say anything, others will start following suit without even knowing that's what you did!

When you let go it makes your whole life better. This includes your health, as demonstrated above. So, take responsibility for your health and environment, and get to work letting go of all the "stuff" with the exercises above. There isn't a "do this every day for thirty days" on this practice to make a habit, because the feeling of relief associated with letting go will be its own reward and will push you to continue doing it. It may take more than one time for the really long-standing history; that's okay and quite common. Continue to do it again and again until it's gone. More things may happen, but the good news is there is not a limit to how many times you can use these exercises, and it becomes easier over time to let go of everything.

CHAPTER 7

REALLY START LISTENING
TO YOURSELF

*"The only thing that matters is: what do I think
of me?"*

– My friend, **Edinne**

O kay, now that you're cooperating with others
to increase your reward pathway in your
brain, feeling grateful, seeing what's right with you,
and letting go of making others responsible for your
health, it's time to start learning what your body
really wants by listening. I'm sure there are many
books that go way more in depth about this, but I

have frequently found myself trying to make a million changes because I feel overwhelmed with suggestions about what to do. I try to make so many changes and cannot sustain them and then give up. I want to make life more simple here and have proven it works through myself and some of my patients. There are also probably a million different ways to accomplish listening more in depth to our bodies that include amazing spiritual retreats and classes, but I would like for you to be able to do it without anybody else's help or having to spend loads of money. Sometimes those extra communities can be wonderful and quite fun, and some of the classes are great if you want to do them. Feel free to further explore them after a base has been created first. If you don't create a base of listening to yourself, then anybody could suggest something and you would start relying again on somebody else to tell you what's right for you. What we are trying to do here is quiet our minds enough to appreciate when a sensation in our body feels abnormal. We all think that we know when we are actually having pain or other symptoms. Sometimes, if we get things like the flu, it is very clear by our fever and sudden vomiting and body aches that we have an illness. I'm not talking about that. I am talking about the chronic illnesses, the subtle changes that snowball over time but are reversible.

Now that we've let go of making somebody else responsible for our health, we can really be honest with ourselves. Maybe we were so busy trying to fix somebody else's life or being angry at somebody else that we ignored our physical symptoms. Maybe we thought that if only we could change our outside situation, then our health would get better. From my experience, things around you don't need to change for you to get better. As an example, I had a patient, let's call him Mark, who was a bus driver. He was on three different medications for high blood pressure and three medications for diabetes. We were getting close to having to start him on insulin because his blood sugar continued to be high even though he was taking all his medications as he was supposed to. Mark was very upset and ready to make a change. We discussed one little change at a time that would help Mark's health. He thought that he would need a different lifestyle and job, and more money to be able to eat better and exercise. We truly only made small changes, but over the following year and a half Mark stopped needing any of his blood pressure or diabetes medication and was healthier than ever. What changes we made are less important than the fact that Mark was ready to change. The changes are also way less important than the fact that Mark took steps to change his thinking before making diet and exercise changes. Overhauling your mind makes it so easy to sustain healthy choices because you learn to love yourself enough to want to keep making healthy choices.

After graduating from residency I began working at a job I loved, doing emergency medicine on rural Native American reservations. I truly enjoyed the Natives who consistently showed more gratitude, appreciation, and joy than any other population I had ever worked with in a city. However, after only a couple of years I began feeling extremely run down. I began having more abnormal heart beats than usual, more migraines, painful sciatica on my right side causing shooting pain down my leg, muscle spasms in the muscles of my spine in my neck, and mid-back increasing chronic pain. I started to look for more things outside of me that would make me feel better, including medications. I started more new medications that didn't seem to work. I tried to do yoga and exercise more. I tried various supplements, better hydration, different forms of exercise. I kept taking everybody else's suggestions and adding things, making caring for myself very complicated and more stressful. I went home wondering why none of this was working because I was "doing everything right according to Western medicine." I was so lucky to meet with some of the Native Americans who lived in the same city as me with the hopes they knew something I didn't know.

I was becoming more stressed out and depressed and the physical pain was not helping. I kept telling them how I felt like I couldn't be what everybody wanted me to be and do what everybody wanted me to do. How I might as well give up because no matter how much I wanted to help I felt like I couldn't do anything right and my body was falling apart. Then one of them said to me, "Stop listening to what everybody else is thinking about you and focus on one thing—what *do you* think of you?" This is something I have kept in my mind ever since. It has empowered me in letting go of listening to every other suggestion and focusing on my needs, not in a selfish way. It helped me know that I am responsible for listening to myself to be able to improve my health. It wasn't until she suggested this that I made actual sustainable changes in my life to improve my health and mood.

I want you to start *only* thinking, "What do I think of me?" Not what does anybody else think. Not, "What does my dad or mom or sister think?" Not, "What will the neighbors or people at church say?" This goes for how we think about other people as well. Too many times I have heard people insulting others out of "concern about them" or "because they love them." Telling somebody they are fat (or insert any insult here) "because you love them" is *not* love. Don't fool yourself into thinking that. Usually what you don't like about them is actually what you don't like about yourself, and that's why you noticed it in them. If you're truly acting out of love with another person you *only* think, "What do *they* think about *themselves?*" and if they are happy, that's it. If they ask you for help, then your job is to fully accept them as you fully accept yourself. To be an example of self-love and make changes out of self-love and not fearing what others say. Changing for somebody else without wanting to change because you love yourself is rarely sustained. I find those that criticize others most are the most hard on themselves, most of the time without recognizing it. My favorite phrase regarding this is, "You spot it, you got it." So, stop picking on others and yourself and think only, "What do I think of me?"

There are certainly people who want to make big physical changes to their body like weight loss, thinking that once their body is better they will feel better both about themselves and physically. The problem that happens is when somebody makes those changes and realize they're still the same person. They can sustain the changes for quite a while, but ultimately seem to go back to their old habits. This is why it is so important to take the steps outlined in this and the previous chapters so that your mind rightfully believes that you deserve to be healthy and happy. Because you do! Everybody deserves to be happy! If you believe that you were born with some horrible body or health and this is how it is and it doesn't get any better, then it's difficult to change and stay changed.

The health benefits of even short meditation have been shown time and time again by science. Now we finally get to start! I'm not talking just improvements in your mood for things like depression and anxiety, which have also been proven, I'm talking about things like every kind of chronic pain.[16] Patients who meditate have a decrease in chronic pain and need less medication, if any. Less medication means fewer side effects that need to be treated by another medication. Even the American Heart Association, the organization that doctors take recommendations from, agrees that meditation may be helpful in decreasing some cardiovascular risks, like heart attack. While there is still a lot of research that needs to be done, at the very least meditation will improve your mood and make life better. It certainly won't hurt you, so give it a real try.[17]

I know I said you don't have to be a guru or meditate eight hours a day to start having better health. However, meditation really is a great place to start. You don't have to believe in God or any sort of religion to gain benefit from being quiet for ten minutes a day. You can actually start with five minutes a day. And guess what? Your mind *is supposed* to wander. That is human nature. The idea is to bring the mind back to whatever you're focusing on—I recommend breath because that's a really easy thing you always have available. You think it won't work for you because you can't pay attention? Guess what? I myself have ADHD and have seen others with ADHD continue to practice and get good at it. Over time with meditation, your mind gets stronger at coming back to what you are focusing on at the beginning. I think this is how meditation helps us most in everyday life. Eventually, with practice bringing my mind back to the breath, I learned to refocus my attention on how well things are going, not all the things wrong with me.

Not everybody wants to do breathing meditation, and quite frankly it was too difficult for me to focus on at the beginning. The great thing is that there are so many various versions of meditation. Walking meditations, guided meditations, even funny meditations you can listen to. I actually love a meditation called honest meditation. If you don't like swearing, please don't listen to this one. You can find it online by searching for "honest meditation," and there is even an app for your phone where you can choose longer meditations if you wish. I use the one by Jason Headley. (No, I don't know him nor am I getting some sort of kickback, though I do imagine he and I would be friends if we met!) I find myself laughing and remembering the point of all of this is not to be serious but to find humor in things. You know how people say laughter is the best medicine? Now, it's proven that laughter delays the onset of heart complications in people with type 2 diabetes.[18] There are many, many other studies and books about the benefits of laughter too. I don't have any one suggestion, but if you're interested I'm sure the internet/your therapist/a trusted friend can help you out.

I quite often suggest ten minutes of meditation daily to my patients. I'm frequently met with the same response: I don't have time. Well, how much time are you spending doing things like taking a medication, picking up the medication, refilling a medication, going to the doctor for the medication? Would you like to not do that? Would you like your overall physical and mental health to get better too? Then find a time. Nobody's going to do it for you. Sometimes I will drive to work without any music on and do my best to take deep breaths the whole way. My goal is to see how long I can pay attention to my breathing. Think of a time you might be alone for ten minutes, then take deep breaths and try to count how many breaths you're taking. That can be enough of a meditation daily to start. I know we all think we have reasons why we don't have time, but guess what? You do.

CHAPTER 8

LESS IS MORE—DIET CHANGES

"Life expectancy would grow by leaps and bounds if green vegetables smelled as good as bacon."
– Doug Larson

Frequently, suicidal patients come into the emergency department. That's where they come to keep safe until we can find a more long-term place for treatment. It is extremely common to feel as if you are alone when you no longer want to live. Patients frequently say to me things like, "You don't know what this is like. I bet you have a perfect life." On more than one occasion I tell them that I myself have felt like not being alive because of depression, and then I will turn to the nurse and ask if they have ever been suicidal or depressed. More often than not, both myself and the nurse taking care of the patient have also felt the same way. I don't mention this because I want sympathy or to make you uncomfortable. I mention this to point out that we are all extremely similar in feeling alone and depressed sometimes. According to the World Health Organization, about seven percent, or one in fourteen U.S. citizens, have experienced a depressive episode *in the past year.* This is steadily increasing from prior years. Additionally, about fifteen percent of the adult population, or one in seven, will experience some serious depression in their lifetime.[19] From what I've seen as a doctor, people just aren't speaking up and getting treatment because of stigma. It's my personal belief that if somebody says that they have never been depressed either they are lying or they just haven't *yet.* I think at some point in everybody's lives they have or will experience some sort of mental health issue. Even if it's not depression, it could be anxiety, fear, trauma…the list is endless.

But why am I talking about depression during the diet chapter? Because every time I have had some depression, I blamed it on having some sort of weak mind. I would beat myself up about how could I not control it and ask myself, "what is wrong with me?" It turns out that every single time I was depressed it was either due to a nutritional problem or a medication side effect causing a nutritional problem. The first time it was a side effect of a medication I was on for the bipolar misdiagnosis that caused my thyroid to be low. The second time it was due to lack of vitamin D, the third time it was due to lack of folate. The second and third time I had also recently had antibiotics that killed the natural bacteria called the microbiome, which I will explain more later in the chapter.

What happens to our diet when we are depressed or anxious or tired? We reach for quick energy or mood boosts in the form of simple carbohydrates. This includes simple sugars and processed grains. When those carbohydrates wear off, our mood crashes leading us to want more carbohydrates. Frequently we beat ourselves up about how we are unable to control our cravings, as if our body is doing something wrong. If you have even a small nutritional deficiency or you're chronically tired like most of America, then your body is appropriately responding by saying it needs quick energy. This becomes a craving for carbohydrates and sugar. So thank your body for craving the appropriate energy source! I, too, have eaten many, many carbohydrates at times when I was exhausted (so basically all of medical school and residency) only to realize I was creating a cycle of needing more carbohydrates to re-balance my mood and get energy back. Ever heard of the term "hangry," being so hungry that you're angry? I've certainly been there and then shoved more sugar in my mouth, usually in the form of fruit, and boom! I'm better. However, it then happens again a couple hours later if I don't supplement with other types of foods to sustain the energy and balance my blood sugar. More to come on that. Now I try to figure out what emotions are going on underneath my eating. I've found it is rarely helpful to tell people (including myself) what they should stop doing. In my opinion, telling somebody what not to eat only makes them want it more. I believe when you add things into your diet that are healthy, your cravings for unhealthy things stop.

I am a believer that your body knows what to do about most types of illness if we give it the right materials and stay out of the way. What do I mean by this? I mean the basic vitamins and minerals along with water. That's right—water. Don't add anything to it, even if you think it's good for you. *Plain water.* Though guidelines vary, a good start for adults is sixty-four ounces per day. So, measure out sixty-four ounces so you know how much that is, and drink at least that. I would recommend filtered water if it's available. The majority of illnesses I see in primary care and the emergency room could be solved with hydration. Things that, if they continue to happen can become chronic illnesses. For example, headaches. Almost every time I see a patient who has a headache, they are not drinking enough water. Without drinking water and then taking things like over-the-counter headache medicine (ibuprofen or acetaminophen), they start down a slippery slope of chronic headache. Any over-the-counter headache medicine can cause rebound headaches when it wears off in four to six hours. Then you need more, which can lead to other, more serious complications. The same thing happens with caffeine. Being dehydrated can cause fatigue, poor sleep, constipation, acne, basically anything.

Have almost any problem? Try water. It's funny to me how many people know the human body is at least sixty percent water, then hardly drink any water throughout the day and wonder why they don't feel well.[20] There is such a thing as too much water though, so if you're feeling constantly thirsty after drinking the minimum amount of water, you should ask your healthcare provider why. As I've said, everything in moderation, and listen to your body.

One note about which diet fad is the best: none of them. If you're going to make changes to your diet, make small changes that you plan on sustaining for the rest of your life. I have seen zero patients who have gone on an extreme diet for some set amount of time and then magically kept healthy eating habits that sustained reversal of their disease. The goal of this whole book is for you to listen to your body about what you need. The simplest way to know the basics of what you should be eating is to imagine that you are a caveman. Was that thing you want to eat around for a caveman? Although I wasn't around during that time, I imagine they mostly ate vegetables, and sometimes whole grains, some lean meats, nuts, fish, and some fruit. Mostly fresh vegetables, though. There is not one thing that is terrible for everybody or one thing that is good for everybody. You are just going to have to figure that out for yourself, by listening to your body. Just keep it as natural as possible, mostly based in vegetables and protein (plant-based or nuts, with occasional meat). Try not to get obsessed with monitoring what you're eating. Being stressed out about what you do and don't eat is a surefire way to create stress, which can ultimately counteract any positive effect of dietary changes. Find moderation and balance. Be gentle with yourself. If you need to review the effects of stress on your body, please refer to Chapter 5.

Remember Mark, the bus driver on many medications for hypertension and diabetes who reversed it all and didn't need medications after one year? After he learned to love himself and felt positive about being able to make small changes, his first change was *adding* food. That's right, he added two cups of sugar snap peas for a month and came back two weeks later saying that he was starting to get dizzy when he stands up. At first I was worried and then we took his blood pressure... it was because he didn't need as many blood pressure medications anymore. I was also astonished since he did not make any other changes in those two weeks.

If you have no dietary restrictions, if I had to choose one thing to add to your diet it would be a raw green vegetable. It can be the same one or a different one every day. You don't have to make a fancy salad or anything—sometimes I just shove raw spinach in my mouth to meet the minimum requirements. Not because I think it's delicious, but because it helps me regulate my diet when I'm too tired to have any willpower about what I'm eating. Which, as a resident and medical student, was all the time. Think you can't afford fresh vegetables? I have noticed that if I start eating two cups of spinach a day my food bill will decrease because I don't get as many cravings for the junk. About two cups per day is all you have to eat. Your blood sugar becomes more stable, meaning a better mood and fewer cravings. With a better mood you are more able to calmly decide which food choices are best for you. So get a bag with two cups of something like celery, broccoli, or spinach, and eat that every day for the rest of your life. Of course vary what it is and don't overdo it. If committing for the rest of your life seems daunting, make a commitment to do it for thirty days. After twenty-one days you'll just want to do it for the rest of your life anyway. If you eat two cups of vegetables and about the same amount of fresh fruit daily you have already decreased your risk for things like heart attack, cancer, and an overall risk of early death.[21]

Earlier in the chapter I mentioned your microbiome. This is all the natural bacteria all over your body, inside and out. There are places that should not have bacteria of course, but those are very few. I talked about how I realized that every time I had some depression I had been on an antibiotic just prior to it. More and more research is confirming that the natural bacteria on and in your body helps to fight many diseases. We need our natural bacteria to help us avoid things like heart disease, cancer, chronic respiratory diseases, stroke, Alzheimer's, diabetes, flu and pneumonia, and kidney disease.[22] My point is although there are definitely times for antibiotics, don't get carried away with thinking they solve everything with no side effects. No antibiotic can target only the certain bacteria causing a problem and have no side effect. There are other medications that can cause an upset in the microbiome other than antibiotics. I would truly recommend at least a temporary probiotic to everybody, whether or not you are taking antibiotics. Try it for thirty days; you know why by now. Even some processed foods can mess with these bacteria that are assisting you in your health. On the package it should say "twenty billion CFUs" and can vary in which type of bacteria. Most are for the gut now, which I think most people need to work on anyway. I think probiotics are ridiculously overpriced, so you can search on the internet to learn about what foods have natural probiotics and see if you can include more in less expensive ways. One great source of probiotic is…fresh vegetables! Which is great because you've already added them now. There are also options like non-dairy yogurt (you can have dairy if you want), fermented foods like kimchi and sauerkraut, and drinks like kombucha. Again, find what's right for you. More expensive does not necessarily mean better.

What are the most basic changes you should make based on this chapter? Drink enough water and eat vegetables, green ones. If you do those two things you will already take care of most things you're missing, including your nutrients and your microbiome. You can try a probiotic if you'd like, but don't break the bank on it if you can eat fruits and vegetables. I would absolutely recommend a probiotic if you have to take an antibiotic for any reason though.

The closer you get back to eating like a caveman, the more your body will naturally have exactly the resources it needs to take care of itself and stay healthy.

The goal for this step is eat at least two cups of green vegetables daily and drink at least sixty-four ounces of *plain water* if you have no dietary/water restrictions. This will get you some changes that will benefit you the rest of your life and stop/reverse chronic diseases before they start. You can (and should) do this for the rest of your life too. You will avoid many expensive trips to the doctor and new medications if you make these small changes. You may even see reversal in as few as two weeks like my patient Mark!

CHAPTER 9

MOVE YOUR BODY

"Exercise is a celebration of what your body can do, not a punishment for what you ate."
– Women's Health UK

As a surgical resident, in the first six months I went up two scrub sizes and gained thirty pounds. I couldn't understand why; I was on my feet all the time working between twelve to sixteen-hour shifts. I knew I didn't have time to get to the gym because I chose to spend more time with my daughter instead, but I thought I was being relatively healthy. Of course I was stressed out, but I did not appreciate how much the lack of sleep was causing problems in my body. I couldn't change my environment or the hours I was working. I tried to find ways to fit in going to the gym, but just could not sustain it. I started paying more attention and realized that I was underestimating how much time I was actually spending sitting or standing still. I knew that I wouldn't be able to undergo some vigorous exercise program, so instead I turned my attention to what I could do while I was at work. Honestly the only big change I really made was only taking stairs. That was it. I was very surprised that I started losing weight almost immediately and the thirty pounds I had gained were gone within four months without any other exercise. This improved my blood sugar, mood, sleep, and back pain almost immediately.

The common idea is that we need to go to the gym or do vigorous exercise for around an hour a day to be healthy or lose weight. I didn't know at the time, but now know that making small activity changes throughout the day can be even better than sitting all day and then going to the gym for an hour. Research has shown that small lifestyle interventions, like taking the stairs or parking your car further away, are just as good as structured exercise programs and in some cases, better.[23] There are studies that even show that getting up and walking around intermittently during the day can help your mood.[24] It can increase concentration and efficiency, so if you're trying to power through something you're working on you will actually get your work done more efficiently and better if you just go on a walk. It doesn't just affect your mind—hopefully I have done my job explaining well enough in this book that when your mood is better, your physical body gets better and vice versa through the habits we create.

There is a phrase that I once heard from a cardiologist I was working with: "exercise begets energy." I guess the original phrase is "energy begets energy," but I liked his version better. What he means by that is you don't one day have all this energy and become ready to exercise. It's the exercise (in the form of movement throughout the day) that then gives you more energy to *want* to do more exercise. There is not going to be one day that you feel motivated to exercise without first doing some exercise. So, if we're learning that moving your body more regularly during the day is as good as exercise at the gym and that increased movement is going to give you more energy, then it's easy to see that little changes make a huge difference. Remember, increased exercise can improve all sorts of chronic illness and is frequently the first recommendation for most diseases. The Mayo Clinic does a wonderful job on their website outlining what an accumulation throughout the day of thirty minutes of high intensity interval training, including just walking briskly, can improve, including but not limited to: asthma, heart disease, arthritis, back pain, dementia, and even cancer.[25]

Maybe you're thinking, "But I don't have anywhere to go walking," and to that I have a few suggestions. Do you have any area you can walk back and forth in, even if it's only five feet long? Then do lunges down the hallway. Do you take bathroom breaks? Do ten to twenty squats each bathroom break. Think of any exercise you can do in your area and do that. I set an alarm for every one to two hours to remind me to get up and do something before exercise became a habit. Remember, it only takes twenty-one days of doing something to make a habit, and then you just do it. I, myself, follow these very same suggestions. Frequently, when working rural emergency medicine I was told that running outside could be dangerous, so I avoided it. Instead, I would do lunges as I walked through the ER to see my next patient. Of course I looked silly and people made fun of me. Keep a good humor about it and laugh, because as we saw earlier in the book, laughter really is scientifically proven medicine! The joke is on them because now you are getting healthy through movement *and* laughter. I find people usually start joining me once I tell them about all of the health benefits. Again, this book is about doing what's right for you and not caring what other people think because you are putting your health first. That includes finding creative ways of getting exercise at work. One of my favorite surgeons to operate with as a resident would stop and make us take a sterile "dance break" where we shook it all out. Of course we made sure it was a safe time to take a break first. My point is to find a way.

Need another example? Remember my patient Mark who was a bus driver for ten hours a day? He would get off the bus and do ten jumping jacks. Of course he was self-conscious at first, but then people started doing them *with* him and it was a fun cooperation (remember, cooperation activates our reward center) with exercise. They would laugh and make it fun. You'll be surprised how much fun people can be if you're unafraid to start the fun.

If you can find time to go walking or exercise outside, even for a moment, you have even more benefit. I have come to find that many jobs are based on being inside and we underestimate how much we actually get outside. We need nature for so many reasons that don't involve it just being beautiful. The health benefits of being outside include improved mood, which is shown to lead to improve blood pressure, decreased muscle tension, better sleep, pretty much everything.[26] Even a plant in a hospital room has been shown to improve outcomes of patients getting surgeries. The sun changes an inactive form of vitamin D to the active form. There are some supplements you can use that may claim to be the active form; however, these aren't proven to be as good as natural sunlight exposure. We need that active form and the best recommendation I could find is a minimum of twenty minutes in the sun each day without sunscreen. I mean straight in the sun, not through any window, since most windows have filters on them. This doesn't mean you need to go all day every day in the sun without sunscreen. Like I said, do what's right for you. I have extremely fair skin—I joke with my daughter that I'm see-through. I have already had a precancerous mole removed from my body. I don't hide from the sun now, I just do it in moderation. Another function of the sun? Decreased dopamine suppression, a fancy way of saying more dopamine, another happiness hormone among other things.[27] You have to let real sunlight into your eyes without staring at the sun. We'll go into this more in the next chapter.

If you feel like you need to look up certain guidelines for exercise, just don't. You don't want to get obsessed or judge yourself for what you're *not* doing and actually sometimes too much exercise can be detrimental for your health (I mean *a lot* of exercise though—this doesn't mean don't exercise). Instead, look at how much a child who does not care yet what people think moves, before we teach them that sitting for long amounts of time is "well-behaved." This is as close to how much our bodies are meant to move as I can guess. I illustrated earlier in this chapter that blocks of exercise weren't as good as moving your body on a regular basis. That doesn't mean that either one is wrong if it's what makes you feel good. Again, make changes you decide are right for you, no matter how small, that you can imagine easily doing for the rest of your life. Then high five yourself for doing it!

The takeaways from this chapter are these: Get up and move your body somehow every one to two hours in whatever way you can. Bonus points if you can laugh while you're doing it. Extra bonus points if you can do it outside sometimes. As above, this is shown to reverse and help you avoid all kinds of chronic disease. It's way easier than you think. It goes without saying, but I'll say it anyway: twenty-one days in a row to make it a habit, but commit to thirty. You'll end up doing it for the rest of your life after you feel how great it is anyway.

CHAPTER 10

WHAT SENSATIONS ARE YOURS?

"A warm smile is the universal language of kindness."

– William Arthur Ward

It was extremely hard for me to grasp how much of the subtle is affecting us in everyday life. My whole life was spent studying things we could see and test. Perhaps I didn't want to believe that there was so much more that we couldn't explain. When people would tell me things were affecting my body that weren't measured in a test with certain facts and statistical analysis I would ignore it completely. I only "worshipped science" that was done in the way I learned was "best practice." Of course when I started doing work as a doctor, I followed what the known "best practice guidelines" were for my patients because that's what I had been taught. Then something happened—I started realizing that maybe this science I was so adamant about may not always be the best possible care. It was ugly. It was basically the adult version of a toddler throwing a tantrum. I was so insistent on believing what I was doing was helping the most every time and no other thing was as good.

How did this realization come about? I have always said that if I could do medical missions for my entire job (meaning go serve the underserved for free) I would. Unfortunately, not only is it uncommon to get paid for medical missions, but physicians pay for them themselves and use rare vacation time (while foregoing spending time with loved ones) simply because they love doing it. With over $300,000 in loans, the bank was not going to allow me to work for free, so I did the next best thing, running around the country fresh out of residency doing the job I loved working in emergency rooms on Native American Reservations. I was also studying for a new board exam in lifestyle medicine because I wanted more sustainable health for my patients than just medications. My plan was to be a kind of Robin Hood of medicine by having those who could pay for treatment help my business stay alive while I gave free treatment to those who truly couldn't afford it. I guess I wanted to be less of a thief and more of a redistribution of wealth center. I had seen that in medical missions when we show up and hand out free medications it might help for a while, but ultimately what happens when the medications run out? I needed to know how I could help people who didn't have access to medications in ways that they could keep up on their own. As I studied more and more lifestyle medicine, I saw the pattern that a lot of the traditional populations had it right already, even though the way it may have been developed and used was based on spiritual traditions and not what doctors call "science."

Around the same time, I met somebody whose job it was to help distribute grants with the Center for Disease Control (CDC) for "Tribal Practices for Wellness in Indian Country." I mentioned this earlier in the book, but the goal was to encourage Native American Tribes to eat and do more activities according to their cultural traditions. There were even studies showing that this helped with diabetes control and may benefit with other diseases. The more I studied the "real science according to doctors," the more I saw we were just proving a lot of the spiritually-based traditions were already right, especially those that were based in loving and respecting ourselves and everybody around us—meaning we are all equal, no matter what.

At the same time it seemed more and more studies were showing that the "scientific recommendations" and medications that I had been prescribing were being found to have side effects as severe as causing cancer. I needed to know more about what "science" was behind what used to be thought of as strictly spiritual practice. Keep in mind that I don't mean religion. I mean truly based in love and compassion for all.

I went over this a bit in a prior chapter, but let's review here. Before I even began to search the literature, I could at least reason out a few things. We take tracings of the heart on a regular basis. What we are measuring is based on the electricity of the heart. We don't see that electricity, but it certainly created something we heavily rely on in medical practice: the EKG. We guide entire treatments in the emergency room based on the electricity of the heart because we found a way to see it with our eyes.

I could then make the link to the research that shows a clear difference in EKG between somebody who is angry and somebody who is appreciative, meaning our feelings actually change this thing we rely on so heavily in the ER.[28] Remember the study I talked about earlier in the book where early research demonstrated that one person detected another's heartbeat without touching? When I was first reading studies about detecting each other, I thought I had slipped into some weird sci-fi realm. Though the research on that is in its early stages and we don't know exactly what it means, it seems to explain a lot in my life, especially about how well I seem to be able to understand others, so much that I seemed to adopt their behaviors and feelings rather quickly. This includes behaviors like anger or stress that had ultimately also led to the physical things I was experiencing on a chronic basis—which were keeping me in need of medications to treat my physical symptoms from the stress.

In psychology, there is a well-known phenomenon called emotional contagion. This is when somebody can adopt how another person feels. There are numerous studies that point to being able to recognize emotions in another person's facial expression, called facial mimicry.[29] However, the same "adoption of emotions" was also found when somebody heard something associated with an emotion, like laughter for example.[30] This is supported by findings like mirror neurons, cells that are located in the brain. These neurons are active just when watching another person do a task. For example, if I watched somebody else do something like pick up a banana, my own brain would have the same activity. I just watched somebody else do an action, which then created the same response in my brain as if I was doing it too. This means that a lot of the overwhelming emotions like stress, fear, and anger that collectively created the chronic physical symptoms I was feeling could possibly have been "picked up" from other people in addition to the stressors in my life. I'm not saying it's responsible for everything, because taking care of my own held-in emotions was necessary for reversal of my chronic diseases. I'm saying through meditation and identifying which things were still bottled in for myself, I was able to start knowing when I was stressed out because of myself or the people around me and letting it go when it wasn't mine more easily.

There are at least two studies that take the banana observation with mirror neurons one step further. One showed that the mirror neurons fired the same when one monkey watched another monkey pick up a banana. After the expected mirror neurons fired the researchers found something very interesting, another specific set of mirror neurons fired based on the intention of what that monkey was going to do. Meaning that the observer could tell what the monkey was going to do next even though he hadn't yet done it, based on the mirror neurons.[31]

What I mean here is that there are numerous studies showing that we don't have to communicate verbally at all to somehow have the same emotions as somebody else and even know their intentions. This truly makes so much sense to me. I will be generally happy and kind to everybody at baseline, but if I get in a group of unhappy people who are mean to each other I become somebody I don't recognize. Throughout my life, I would continually beat myself up for not being kind and calm in every situation, but I was adopting behaviors and attitudes that I knew I did not have when I was alone. When I learned about all of this research, and with some help from my friends, I realized how much the unseen really was affecting me. How maybe it was not just the folate and vitamin D deficiency and some lack of mental strength causing such emotional difficulty, leading to physical problems, but I was around suicidal patients every time I worked, and my emotions mirrored that. I also learned that perhaps I couldn't blame everybody else's actions or negativity just on themselves, but perhaps, without knowing it, they were "detecting me." I had to address my feelings inside, too.

Since then I have been doing even more meditation to understand what it feels like for me to be alone so that when I'm around groups of people I can recognize what it is I'm feeling. I do this by being as calm as possible and then recalling events when I felt angry, happy, etc., with the help of the book I mentioned before, *The Language of Emotions* by Karla McLaren. I try to experience almost every emotion while alone so I can be myself and identify them as physical sensations. For example, when I'm anxious I know I get really tense shoulders, and instead of trying to fight against being anxious, I listen to what my anxiety is telling me. Every emotion is there for a reason after all, and I believe we keep on feeling it until we recognize and remedy the problem. If I'm feeling some sort of strong emotion around other people, I take a deep breath and try to get my body to feel how calm I know I can feel during meditation. This is why meditation is so important, so we can return to our original state and not act out according to somebody else's emotions. When two people are arguing and it's going back and forth and escalating, it seems to me to be two people actually taking on the others' feelings, but if you know which are yours then it's easier to stop and take a breath. Then, when you are away from the situation, you can deal with your own emotions and not continually blame somebody else.

We already established that emotions affect our bodies, so once I got at least a little handle on which feelings were mine and how to recognize and release them, almost all of my chronic medical issues started improving. I started getting fewer and fewer migraines, my back pain and sciatica started improving, and I started to feel better. I had more energy because I could easily let go of what wasn't mine that was shown to cause fatigue. For example, another person's depression or anxiety could exhaust me if I didn't realize I was carrying it around. That, mixed with your own emotions, can create problems for your whole body if you're not careful.

Not everybody feels all of this at the same level, which I didn't know at first. People would say "you're too sensitive" and I would feel terrible about myself, like somehow I was weak or something was wrong with me. Now, though, I try to laugh because, generally speaking, the people who are saying that to me are those with the most uncomfortable feelings inside. They don't like my sensitivity because they can't even deal with their own feelings, so mine become uncomfortable and almost foreign, especially when I am very kind and accepting or have an optimistic attitude. That doesn't mean something is wrong with them, it just means they've learned to do things another way. Let me put that into an example—it's as if we learned different languages as children and now the two of us must perform an emergency surgery on an unconscious patient. One of us does anesthesia while the other is a surgeon; different skills, but both needed for the well-being of the patient. We don't sit around and get mad at each other because the other's skill is different or they speak another language—that is a waste of time and energy. If we did that, the patient would just lie there and die. Nothing was wrong with the language each of us learned, but now instead of continually pointing that out, we learn to use our strengths to get the task done.

Say we were successful and the patient did well, everybody is happy. Just like the analogy, I know that my skill set of sensitivity has been such a huge gift with my patients—even when I'm being criticized by others—and that's what matters to me most.

CHAPTER 11

WHEN DO I GET OFF THE MEDS?

"The doctor of the future will give no medicine, but will interest her or his patients in the care of the human frame, in a proper diet, and in the cause and prevention of disease."

– Thomas Edison

I know you've been reading this book wondering, "When is she going to give me some practical advice for exactly how to taper off of my medication?" And I must emphasize that just stopping your medicine can be extremely dangerous, so please work with a professional to taper off safely when you're ready. Make sure you also understand exactly what can happen if you come off of the medication. Sometimes medications are keeping you alive, so don't just throw them out if they are necessary.

I am certainly hoping by now that you can understand there is no one-size-fits-all. I can't say for everybody how quickly or slowly you should come off a medication, just like I can't recommend the same medication to every patient. I can tell you that the more work you put into being healthier, the easier it is to come off of your medications. The whole point is for you to stop looking at your body as something so wrong and to start appreciating what so right with it. It is not until you see what's right that you start letting go of what's wrong. It took me a long time to realize that my particular skill sets were not the same as every other doctor's, and thank goodness they weren't, because if we all had the same skill sets and interests we would all be the same type of doctor! As I talked about earlier, that goes for the whole population: if we all knew exactly the same thing then how would we all be working together to sustain life? Nothing would work if we all were a doctor or a plumber, or any other job. We all matter because we all have a role to play that is unique to ourselves, even if not just in our job.

I know that I say quite frequently to listen to what's right for you, and I agree that is the most important thing. I cannot tell you how many times I have asked a patient what they thought was wrong and, if they really thought about it, they were usually right. The key there is *they* thought about it, on their own with the information they had. They didn't base their opinion on what the internet or other people were telling them. The problem is when we blindly believe everything we see. Remember the line from *Sex and the City* where Miranda says, "I just type in my symptoms online and wait for cancer to pop up"? You can create fear and sadness over just about anything if you look for ways to confirm it. What I mean is it's really easy to be scared if you are online looking at the worst possible thing that you might have! I don't think it's bad to look online or in books for what might be causing something. Just spend *more time* finding out the free changes you can make in your life to improve it. The things you can do for yourself that are not putting something into your body or paying for something. The *free* stuff that creates a lifetime of positive change. Then, take it to your doctor, but this time you can have a discussion about what you can do to make it better. You've explored your options that maybe even your doctor don't know about. As discussed before, doctors are, after all, only human and don't know everything. We wish we did, but that's impossible for anybody, even after spending most of our lives studying and doing it. Things are constantly changing, and new options are always coming up. It would take more than the time in a day to know about all of them.

One note about screens (including TV, computers, handheld devices, etc.) while we are on the topic. While I wouldn't recommend staring directly at the sun, don't hide from it like a vampire behind sunglasses. One study found that when our eyes have light hitting them, melatonin is suppressed, which leads to more dopamine. Some of the structures of our eyes are responsible for this regulation of melatonin based on exposure to light.[32] But don't we need melatonin to sleep? Yes! When your eye is no longer exposed to light, your brain will no longer decrease your melatonin level.

The next thing I'm going to say is extremely difficult for most of us, including me, so make sure you're sitting when you read this. The light hitting the eye suppressing our melatonin means our screens are contributing to insomnia. Any screen. Your body can't tell if you're in "night mode" or whatever. It is *exquisitely* sensitive to this, so stop with the screens at least two hours before bedtime—totally. Just because you use screens less doesn't mean they don't do the exact same thing or somehow you're immune. If you're making up a reason why you *need to* check your screen, then let me clarify something for you: your body does not care what this reason is. It will keep on doing the same thing, and good thing! That means your body is behaving exactly as it should, not based on what other people think it should do.

I don't think Western medicine is evil. Everything in moderation is the key. When you need something because your safety or the safety of others is threatened, then use it. The most recent data from the World Health Organization is, "The lifetime risk of maternal death in high-income countries is one in 3,300, compared to one in forty-one in low-income."[33] Childbirth is described here because it is a well-studied medical topic, but this can be true for a lot of medical issues, especially those we don't have much control over. While there may certainly be more than one reason to explain this, Western medicine is absolutely a part of it. I think that natural childbirth is wonderful and admire the women who can do it. They seem to recover faster afterwards. However, when childbirth is not going well and there are signals (like a dropping heart rate) that a baby will die if they don't get out, then it's time to intervene with these interventions these women in low-income countries don't have. Why? Because they don't have Western medicine (among other things).

Believe me, I would absolutely love for every person to have a natural childbirth where both they and the baby survived and were healthy. I believe most doctors do. I would certainly hope every doctor allows for a patient to be as natural as they wish and don't force a C-section on somebody. I love that midwives and doulas exist to be there more during the process of labor and coach women through, because as much as we want to be there with every patient, we can't because we must handle the emergencies. However, if you aren't progressing and they are worried about if the baby is safe, where do you go? The hospital, because without another form of intervention, usually Western medicine, more mothers and babies die.

Should we give medications and perform surgeries on *every* patient? No, of course not. Few doctors want to cut open another person "for fun" because we know all the risks we are taking. I'm saying if there's an emergency, thank goodness we have Western medicine. I have heard of patients literally saying, "I want to have my baby among the lily pads and just keep on with my day like they do in Africa." When I tell this to my actual African patients, they look at me like, "Is she nuts? That is absolutely not what happens!" This demonstrates the problem of just believing what somebody is saying without doing your own research. There is a place for all forms of childbirth and some people prefer not to experience the pain while knowing the risks. Which way is right? Whatever you choose, but remember, if your choice is right for you then the other person's choice is right for them, too.

Childbirth is also a great analogy for almost any other illness that can be treated with Western medicine. You get to choose whether or not to use the medication, but natural childbirth does involve an appropriate amount of pain. I say "appropriate" because there is an amount of pain involved in everything worth doing, it seems. It is a little "painful" for me to get up and move my body when I want to sit around all day— mostly in the form of emotional pain, but sometimes physically. However, later on this results in *less* pain physically. The reason I get up and move my body is because I want to give my body its most natural and optimal state. In turn, my body is able to take care of the functions it is already able to do that keep me from needing medications. Sometimes something may not be as literal as an immediate threat to my life, but may still warrant an "emergency" medication like an antibiotic or I will eventually die from it. I take it for the amount of time prescribed and do everything I can to restore my natural health. I use the medication I need for the least amount of time, but find out what's underneath as to why I needed it and make what changes I can to prevent it in the future. For example, high blood sugar leads to more infections that need antibiotics. If I need the antibiotic to save my life, I take it while evaluating what I need to change to avoid it again in the future.

Everybody can do this, but what you must do first is accept that improving health, like any aspect life, is not beautiful, wonderful, and easy all the time—but it's certainly worth it. There are difficult diseases to counteract but that means that the reward is even greater. Even if our parents and grandparents had the same disease, most times this does not mean we *must* have it. There are very few illnesses that just happen to us and that we have no control over. So know your choices, choose to better yourself, and choose to believe that you *can* change your health, because it's more true than you think! As soon as you know that you're halfway there.

I know it feels like your doctor does not have the time to answer all your questions. As a doctor I also want to spend more time with my patients. It is a very broken system we have that needs some serious fixing when doctors and patients want to spend more time together but can't. That will take some time though. In the meantime, you can get more from your appointment by answering some questions ahead of time. One of the proven ways a doctor will help a patient change is something called "motivational interviewing," which is basically letting the patient decide which changes they will make. When you think about what you want to change, start very small at the beginning, with something you *know* you can change forever (not just for a few weeks) for lifelong health. Then you can move on to bigger goal setting later. I've created some questions with my own modifications below to use as a talking point so less time is spent on questions and more on formulating a plan together! This way you will be working together as a team to make decisions.

Which disease/problem do you dislike the most?

What are all the great things your body is doing correctly?

Which medication (just one for now) do you dislike the most?

How much *plain water* are you drinking in ounces? If you don't know, look at a water bottle. It says ounces on it. Then guess! Keep track of how many of those you drink daily.

How many cups of *plain/raw* vegetables are you eating daily? What kind?

What is your understanding about how the disease occurred in your body?

What is your understanding about what changes in your everyday life would reverse the disease (not the endpoint, a change you make every day)?

Which of these changes are you willing to try?

Which *one* of these would be the easiest for you to do, that you can say with certainty you can absolutely accomplish? (Make *one* easily attainable goal that you can sustain for the rest of your life. If you aren't sure of any of them, then find a creative goal that fits your needs. You can set more in the future if you aren't sure this is enough.)

Imagine that you have made this change a permanent part of your life. How do you feel? (When it is hard to continue the change, remember how it will feel so you can keep going.)

Who can support you in this change in your life? Have you talked to them about it? Would they like to make the change with you? (It's not required but can sometimes be more fun and sustainable this way.)

What is a healthy free reward you can give yourself for doing this thing every day?

CHAPTER 12

NOW IT'S YOUR TURN

*"The impediment to action advances the action.
That which stands in the way becomes the way."*
– Marcus Aurelius

I have a journal somebody gave me that has a saying on it: "Love yourself and everything else falls into place." I used to roll my eyes at this all the time, thinking it was some phrase you put on an inspirational poster and wasn't an actual way people felt. It turns out that it is totally right. I believe that this also applies to diseases and Western medicine. When you're ready to make the changes it becomes much easier if you love yourself first and then actively surround yourself with other people making those changes. So recruit all your friends and family to do it with you! It's a free adventure you can all do together. High five each other and yourself! Point out how much the other person is doing right! Remember that your happiness is contagious to others, proven by science. Don't wait for somebody to make the change first though, because now you know exactly what to do.

I hope you've seen here that the real ability to reverse disease and come off medication starts with believing that you can do it. There are many clichés about acting your way into better thinking. I tried so hard my entire life to think my way into feeling better mentally and physically. It wasn't until I shut off my mind and took action that things became easier, I became healthier, and I was able to come off of my medications. Here were the cheapest/most free actions I could find to do it. I know there are some people that cannot, at least right now, do all of this, so do the best you can.

Taking action includes:

- Cooperating with others through things like anonymous random acts of kindness or just showing compassion to somebody having a bad day. (This activates the reward center of the brain, even if there is no tangible payoff, and increases the likelihood of further cooperation, leading to more reward and feelings of happiness.)

- Actually physically making lists of what's right with you and what you're grateful for. (Proven to increase happiness, not the other way around. Meaning you don't get happy *first* and then grateful, you get grateful first then happy.)

- Meditation of any sort for ten minutes a day. (Increases focus, mood, attitude, and sleep while it decreases anxiety and depression: all of this leading to better blood sugar, less pain, and improved overall physical health as well.)

- Moving your body throughout the day. (Increases concentration/focus, mood, sleep, regulates blood sugar, and is better than sitting around then going to the gym, *and* gives you more energy.)

- Getting in nature/direct sunlight. (Iamproves mood, sleep, blood sugar, vitamin D, and so much more.)

- Laughing. (Shown to delay heart conditions in people with diabetes and of course much more.)

- Eating two cups of fresh green vegetables a day. (I can't even list all the benefits, but basically makes everything better including mood/sleep. Will help decrease your cravings for other food.)
- Hydrate with plain water, filtered if possible, about sixty-four ounces a day if you're an adult with no water restrictions. (See your doctor if you have any questions.)
- Stop any screens two hours before bedtime.
- Use questions in Chapter 11 to guide specific medication conversations with your doctor.

This book was meant to help others see the free and easy ways to decrease their need for medication by getting healthier for life. I intentionally started with helping others and appreciating your own body. If studying the human body rigorously for many years has taught me anything, it is that the human body is extraordinary. Even a body with multiple diseases is doing so many things right that we can't see all the time. It may seem a little too positive to make that leap, so start small. For example, it is quite complicated how and when the body breathes, despite us having no idea it is happening. It speeds up and slows down based on small exchanges of molecules and imbalances. It is controlled by a complex cooperation between our brain, kidneys, blood, small molecules in our bloodstream, electrolytes, cells, blood vessels, air exchange…basically every system of our body plays a role in regulating our breathing, yet it goes on without us having to think about it. That is pretty amazing to me. So, if you're breathing, your body is coordinating a whole lot more than just air in and out.

It's time to stop being angry at what's going wrong in our bodies, because that is making our diseases worse. Give your body a break! Thank it for continuing to function despite our insults to it both emotionally and physically. When I'm starting to get mad at my body because of pain or any other problem, I'm reminded of something I saw once, a video where women were interviewed about what they hated about themselves. They spoke about various physical flaws like being too fat or too thin, having acne or bad hair, really beating themselves up. Then the women were shown pictures of themselves when they were children and asked, "Would you talk to this child that way?" Every single one of them started crying realizing how mean they were to themselves. I think it's time we start talking to our bodies and ourselves the way we would talk to a child we love. I know some people don't like kids, but just imagine a person or a pet you would never talk to like that. Think about how you would instead talk to that person or pet, how you would more likely encourage the good parts of them. If that's not how you would talk to a child, then try to understand why you feel like you have to criticize. I felt that way before, like the only way to improve was to criticize myself until I changed. Because I criticized myself so much, I criticized others too. It took over thirty years for me to see that this does not create better health and happiness. I know for some it is still ongoing, for most or all of their lives, so I feel extremely lucky I learned it at a relatively young age.

It was very uncomfortable to make that change because it felt so unnatural to be kind to myself. I loved encouraging my patients, though. It was so easy to have compassion for those I was helping, but I couldn't sustain kindness to others without learning to give it to myself first. Over time (and it's still a work in progress) I applied that same kind of thinking to myself. Some days it does not come naturally but everything seems to get a little easier and more fun when I try. I start feeling better physically and reach for medications less and less, even on bad days. If you don't think it will work for you then turn off your brain and take action. Like I said, it's much easier to act ourselves into better thinking than vice versa. You've got this.

ACKNOWLEDGMENTS

Thank you to Angela Lauria and The Author Incubator's team, as well as to David Hancock and the Morgan James Publishing team for helping me bring this book to print.

THANK YOU!

Thank you so much for reading my book! If you're interested in further work with me please inquire at reinharttaylormd@gmail.com or on my webpage, DrReinhartTaylor.com. I am available to do telemedicine for clients from anywhere in the world. Thank you again and I look forward to hearing from you.

ABOUT THE AUTHOR

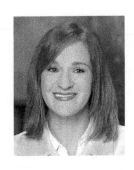

Dr. Rachel Taylor is a board-certified family medicine physician and member of the American College of Lifestyle Medicine with a passion for underserved population work. During her medical mission work she desired to find ways that populations could be treated without medication. Over time she was able to use her experience to help both herself and her patients improve without medications. She has now made it her mission to help stop and reverse diseases using her unique knowledge of combining Western medicine with practical lifestyle changes.

ENDNOTES

1   https://www.chronicdisease.org/page/
    whyweneedph2imphc
2   ADA Website: http://www.diabetes.org/advocacy/
    news-events/cost-of-diabetes.html
3   Liu C, Zhang Y, Jiang H, Wu H (2017)
    Association between social support and post-
    traumatic stress disorder symptoms among
    Chinese patients with ovarian cancer: A multiple
    mediation model. PLoS ONE 12(5): e0177055.
    https://doi.org/10.1371/journal.pone.0177055
4   Katharina Gapp1,3, Johannes Bohacek1,
    Jonas Grossmann2, Andrea M Brunner1,4,
    Francesca Manuella1, Paolo Nanni2 and Isabelle

M Mansuy*, Potential of Environmental Enrichment to Prevent Transgenerational Effects of Paternal Trauma, Neuropsychopharmacology (2016) 41, 2749–2758

5   Morren MA, Przybilla B, Bamelis M, Heykants B, Reynaers A, Degreef H. Atopic dermatitis: triggering factors. J Am Acad Dermatol. 1994;31:467–473

6   Kendra K. Kattelmann, Kibbe Conti, Cuirong Ren. "The Medicine Wheel Nutrition Intervention: A Diabetes Education Study with the Cheyenne River Sioux Tribe." *Journal of the American Dietetic Association*, 2009; 109 (9): 1532 DOI: 10.1016/j.jada.2009.06.362 Jamie Stang. Improving Health among American Indians through Environmentally-Focused Nutrition Interventions. *Journal of the American Dietetic Association*, 2009; 109 (9): 1528 DOI: 10.1016/j.jada.2009.06.371

7   Sonja Nisslé & Tom Bschor (2002) Winning the jackpot and depression: Money cannot buy happiness, International Journal of Psychiatry in Clinical Practice, 6:3, 183-186, DOI: 10.1080/136515002760276144

8   https://www.forbes.com/sites/ duncanmadden/2019/03/28/ranked-the-

10-happiest-countries-in-the-world-in-
2019/#18ad8d6d48a5

9 http://www.thedarwinproject.com/revolution/
revolution.html

10 WIREs Cogn Sci 2016, 7:59–71. doi: 10.1002/
wcs.1377

11 Fenton JJ, Jerant AF, Bertakis KD, Franks P.
The Cost of Satisfaction: A National Study of
Patient Satisfaction, Health Care Utilization,
Expenditures, and Mortality. *Arch Intern
Med.* 2012;172(5):405–411. doi:10.1001/
archinternmed.2011.1662

12 Britta Wilms, Rodrigo Chamorro, Manfred
Hallschmid, Denisa Trost, Nelli Forck, Bernd
Schultes, Matthias Mölle, Friedhelm Sayk,
Hendrik Lehnert, Sebastian M Schmid,
Timing Modulates the Effect of Sleep Loss on
Glucose Homeostasis, *The Journal of Clinical
Endocrinology & Metabolism*, Volume 104, Issue
7, July 2019, Pages 2801–2808, https://doi.
org/10.1210/jc.2018-02636
Spiegel, Karine et al. "Impact of sleep debt on
metabolic and endocrine function." *The Lancet*
354 (1999): 1435-1439.

13 Progress in Neuro-Psychopharmacology and
Biological Psychiatry. DNA methylation
correlates of PTSD: Recent findings and technical

challenges Filomene G.Morrison, Mark W.Miller, Mark W.Logue, Michele Assefe Erika J.Wolf. Volume 90, 2 March 2019, Pages 223-234

14 The Effects of Emotions on Short-Term Power Spectrum Analysis of Heart Rate Variability By: Rollin McCraty, Mike Atkinson, William Tiller, Glenn Rein and Alan D. Watkins. *The American Journal of Cardiology*, Volume 76, NO 14, Noverber 15, 1995, Pages 1089-1093

15 McCraty, R., Atkinson, M.J., Tomasino, D.E., & Tiller, W.A. (2002). "The Electricity of Touch: Detection and Measurement of Cardiac Energy Exchange Between People."

16 Zeidan, F. and Vago, D. R. (2016), "Mindfulness meditation–based pain relief: a mechanistic account." Ann. N.Y. Acad. Sci., 1373: 114-127. doi:10.1111/nyas.13153

17 "Meditation and Cardiovascular Risk Reduction: A Scientific Statement from the American Heart Association." *J Am Heart Assoc.* 2019;8(2):e004176. Published 2019 Jan 15. doi:10.1161/JAHA.117.004176

18 "Homeostatic effect of laughter on diabetic cardiovascular complications: The myth turned to fact", Noureldein, Mohamed H. et al. Diabetes Research and Clinical Practice, Volume 135, 111—119

19 https://www.who.int/news-room/fact-sheets/ detail/depression

20 Mitchell HH, Hamilton TS, Steggerda FR, Bean HW. The Chemical Composition of The Adult Human Body and Its Bearing on the Biochemistry of Growth. J. Biol. Chem. 1945 158: 625.

21 1.Aune D, Giovannucci E, Boffetta P, et al. Fruit and Vegetable Intake and The Risk of Cardiovascular Disease, Total Cancer and All-Cause Mortality-A Systematic Review and Dose-Response Meta-Analysis of Prospective Studies. *Int J Epidemiol.* 2017;46(3):1029–1056. doi:10.1093/ije/dyw319. 2.Blekkenhorst LC, Sim M, Bondonno CP, et al. Cardiovascular Health Benefits of Specific Vegetable Types: A Narrative Review. *Nutrients.* 2018;10(5):595. Published 2018 May 11. doi:10.3390/nu10050595

22 Whole Body Microbiome. Book by Jessica Findlay PhD.

23 JAMA. 1999 Jan 27;281(4):327-34. Comparison of Lifestyle and Structured Interventions to Increase Physical Activity and Cardiorespiratory Fitness: A Randomized Trial. Dunn AL1, Marcus BH, Kampert JB, Garcia ME, Kohl HW 3rd, Blair SN.

24 Sitting-Time, Physical Activity, and Depressive Symptoms in Mid-Aged Women van Uffelen, Jannique G.Z. et al. American Journal of Preventive Medicine, Volume 45, Issue 3, 276—281

25 https://www.mayoclinic.org/healthy-lifestyle/fitness/in-depth/exercise-and-chronic-disease/art-20046049

26 Berman, M. G., Jonides, J., & Kaplan, S. (2008). The Cognitive Benefits of Interacting with Nature. *Psychological Science, 19*(12), 1207-1212
Bowler, D. E., Buyung-Ali, L. M., Knight, T. M., & Pullin, A. S. (2010). A Systematic Review of Evidence for The Added Benefits to Health of Exposure to Natural Environments. *BMC Public Health, 10,* 456.
Bringslimark, T., Patil, G., & Hartig, T. (2008). The Association Between Indoor Plants, Stress, Productivity and Sick Leave in Office Workers. *Acta Horticulturae, 775,* 117.
Devries, S. (2003). "Natural Environments—Healthy Environments? An Exploratory Analysis of The Relationship Between Greenspace and Health." *Environment and Planning, 35*(10), 1717.
Hu, Z. (2008). Linking Stroke Mortality with Air Pollution, Income, and Greenness in Northwest

Florida: An Ecological Geographical Study. *International Journal of Health Geographics, 7*, 1.

Kim, T. (2010). Human Brain Activation in Response to Visual Stimulation with Rural and Urban Scenery Pictures: A Functional Magnetic Resonance Imaging Study *Science of the Total Environment, 408*(12), 2600.

Diette, G. B., Lechtzin, N., Haponik, E., Devrotes, A., & Rubin, H. R. (2003). Distraction Therapy with Nature Sights and Sounds Reduces Pain During Flexible Bronchoscopy: A Complementary Approach to Routine Analgesia. *Chest, 123*(3), 941-948.

Dijkstra, K., Pieterse, M., & Pruyn, A. (2006). Physical Environmental Stimuli That Turn Healthcare Facilities into Healing Environments Through Psychologically Mediated Effects: Systematic Review. *Journal of Advanced Nursing, 56*(2), 166-181.

27 Light, Dark, and Melatonin: Emerging Evidence for The Importance of Melatonin in Ocular Physiology R Brennan, J E Jan & C J Lyons *Eye* volume 21, pages 901–908 (2007)

28 The Effects of Emotions on Short-Term Power Spectrum Analysis of Heart Rate Variability By: Rollin McCraty, Mike Atkinson, William Tiller, Glenn Rein and Alan D. Watkins The American

Journal of Cardiology, Volume 76, NO 14, November 15, 1995, Pages 1089-1093

29 Hatfield, Elaine et al. New Perspectives on Emotional Contagion: A Review of Classic and Recent Research on Facial Mimicry and Contagion. "Interpersona: An International Journal on Personal Relationships," [S.l.], v. 8, n. 2, p. 159-179, dec. 2014. ISSN 1981-6472. Available at: https://interpersona.psychopen.eu/article/view/162. Date accessed: 12 aug. 2019. doi: http://dx.doi.org/10.5964/ijpr.v8i2.162.

30 Hietanen, J. K., Surakka, V., & Linnankoski, I. (1998). Facial Electromyographic Responses to Vocal Affect Expressions. *Psychophysiology, 35*, 530-536.

31 Iacoboni M, Molnar-Szakacs I, Gallese V, Buccino G, Mazziotta JC, Rizzolatti G. Grasping the Intentions of Others with One's Own Mirror Neuron System. PLoS Biol. 2005; 3:e79. 2. Fogassi L, Ferrari PF, Gesierich B, Rozzi S, Chersi F, Rizzolatti G. Parietal lobe: From action organization to intention understanding. Science. 2005; 308: 662–7.

32 Review| Published: 22 September 2006 Light, Dark, and Melatonin: Emerging Evidence for the Importance of Melatonin in Ocular Physiology

R Brennan, J E Jan & C J Lyons *Eye* volume 21, pages 901–908 (2007)

33 https://data.unicef.orgtopic/maternal-health/maternal-mortality/